Pebbling the Walk

Surviving Cancer Caregiving

Pebbling the Walk
Surviving Cancer Caregiving

Steve Reed

Blue Heron Publishing
Portland, Oregon

Pebbling the Walk: Surviving Cancer Caregiving
By Steve Reed

Copyright © 2000 by Stephen C. Reed

Blue Heron Publishing
420 SW Washington Street, Suite 303
Portland, OR 97204
(503) 221-6841
www.BlueHeronPublishing.com

Blue Heron Publishing is a division of A-Concept, Inc.

Cover design by Sue Tencza.
Interior design and production by Martha Ruttle.

ISBN 0-936085-63-0

Printed and bound in the United States of America on pH-balanced paper.

First edition, August 2000
9 8 7 6 5 4 3 2 1

Dedication

This is dedicated to my wife Marthy, who intends to live and laugh forever. And to my brother Chris and sister Karen, who are sitting somewhere up there laughing and saying, "So you thought you were going to write the Great American Novel."

Acknowledgement

The publication of this book was made possible by a generous grant from the King County Arts Commission. The author and publisher thank the Commission for its support.

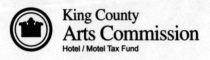

King County
Arts Commission
Hotel / Motel Tax Fund

Contents

Foreword

Although there are hundreds of books written for cancer patients undergoing treatment, there are few books written specifically for caregivers. *Pebbling the Walk* addresses the impact of cancer treatment on both the patient and caregiver—as well as the relationship between them—in an unfalteringly direct, yet joyful way.

Steve Reed has a great deal of experience as a caregiver for the terminally ill. He helped two of his siblings battle lymphoma, and he cared for his wife through her treatment for breast cancer. He also has served as caregiver for other family members—his aunt, mother, and stepfather. In *Pebbling the Walk*, Reed draws from these experiences and uses his wisdom, empathy, and best of all, his humor to write about both the day-to-day tasks of caregiving, like feeding a patient and managing medications, and the more philosophical concerns of caregivers themselves.

Pebbling the Walk is an important book for anyone who has a loved one undergoing cancer treatment. The book's message is powerful and simple: love and laughter can sustain patients and caregivers through even the worst cancer treatment and the uncertainty of life after that treatment. Reed has filled this book with both pragmatic and playful suggestions—including exercises at the end of each chapter—which can significantly elevate the spirits of both patients and caregivers. Many of the suggestions are simply based on common sense, which can be lost in the stress of cancer treatment. Other suggestions are truly inspired and exceedingly helpful. Some suggestions may seem silly at first, but they will probably do the most to lighten the spirit. Caregivers and patients should try these exercises: there is no question that they will help.

Above all, *Pebbling the Walk* is intriguing and heartwarming because Reed is able to discuss common frustrating concerns in a way that brings them down to earth and allows caregivers to realize that they are not only surmountable, but also constructive. This book gives caregivers the tools to better care for their patients and transform cancer treatment into an opportunity to grow and develop a new appreciation for life.

Leah deRoulet, M.S.W.
Social Work Supervisor
Tumor Institute
Swedish Medical Center
Seattle, WA

Preface

I nearly titled this book *One Eye Weeping* because, as an odd aside to the extensive chemotherapy Marthy underwent, one of her eyes would often weep without apparent cause (usually the right eye). Her mood never appeared to be the reason; even at times when she might be happiest, tears could spontaneously flow down one cheek. The depiction of a single eye weeping, as impossibly metaphorical as one hand clapping, seemed representative of the phenomenon that is chemotherapy.

I'm glad I didn't title it that. Such a title would have lent a maudlin atmosphere to the book. Tears are not what this book is about. This book is about happiness, not sadness. What we need are both eyes laughing, even while the tears stream from one or the other, even while the darkest of hours plays around us. All of us, regardless of whether we battle for our lives immediately or not, must live as if there were no more tomorrows, laugh as if there were no more jokes, and love as if there were no more hearts. Each of us is the last of ourselves. After us, we will be no more.

So I wrote this book not about weeping but about celebrating, especially if you find yourself a caregiver to someone struggling to live. If you're a caregiver and you don't know how to dance, get ready to learn. If you're a cancer patient, you are also welcome to read this book, but be sure to give it to your caregiver. There are enough books for cancer patients. This book is for caregivers.

Many thanks to all of you who contributed stories of your treatments, cures, and failures. To those who are still alive, hip-hip-hooray! To those who are not, see you soon raccoons. This book does not intend or pretend to stay the reaper; everyone dies, just as everyone eats. It's up to you whether you mouth oatmeal or feast on the finest cuisine—bon appetite.

Chapter One

If You're Not Laughing, You're Not Living

Poet Rick Fields, experiencing stage-four lung cancer, said that it occurred to him that he didn't have a life-threatening disease, but a disease-threatening life. So it should be for each of us, whether we fight a deadly cancer or simply struggle to rise each morning smiling. We stumble through life hiding from our ultimate demise. Death, it has been said, is the great equalizer. But we all die. Why do we fear it more than some tragedies that happen to only a select few, like blindness, amputation, paralysis, or mental illness? There are certainly fates worse than death, yet we fear the Grim Reaper more than anything else.

It is our fear of what ultimately concludes our lives that determines the very quality of them. The key, of course, is not to fear death. We must invert our perspective as Rick Fields has. Our lives are not threatened by death, but rather the reverse is true. Our deaths must be threatened by our lives.

As my little brother Chris battled his lymphoma, he often broke into laughter at the blackest and most challenging times of his treatment. I'd ask him what he found so funny. He'd shake his head and say, "Sometimes it gets so bad that all you can do is laugh."

He reminds me of the namesake character in *Zorba the Greek*. When Zorba has failed his employer and friend and all is lost, he begins a madcap dance. The employer is astounded and asks him how he can dance at such a time. Zorba replies that sometimes, the only thing a person *can* do is dance.

Sometimes life gets so bad all a person can do is laugh. Throw your head back and spit in the eye of the Universe. Your gesture doesn't change anything but your perspective, but your perspective changes everything.

Chris was the inveterate practical joker before he was diagnosed with cancer. He was also a professor at an Ivy League school, which offered him a droll backdrop for many of his pranks. His humor never waned after he began his prolonged battle; rather, it blossomed into something his associates at times deemed unholy. As his battle was slowly lost, his sense of humor grew stronger rather than weaker. When times were darkest, when all around him felt crushed under the weight of our grief, he lightened our spirits with his jokes and wit.

Chris had to be his own advocate then; I was a neophyte caregiver and was unable to see past my own loss, my own selfish desire to save him. I sat dourly by as he failed, weighing him down further with my fears.

"Humor," he reminded me, "may be the only true art of living." Then I'd find the toothpaste in my tube replaced with shaving cream.

My sister Karen fell to the same lymphoma a few years later. Her fight was particularly difficult because she helped care for our brother as he failed and knew too well what lay ahead for herself. Mercifully, she succumbed in one short year where our brother had struggled for five. As aggressive as her lymphoma proved to be, as painful and frightening, she never lost her sense of humor either. She admonished us all to maintain ours, even to the end.

In her last hours she lay in her bed overlooking her forested yard. I looked up at the trees above us, my eyes filling, my heart breaking.

"Sis," I said, "I love you more than, than your maples have leaves, more than your firs have needles."

She laughed at me.

"You're so full of it," she said.

After her passing, I cared for other family members: a stepfather who died of five different kinds of cancer, an aunt who passed with a stroke, another aunt who died of Alzheimer's, and now my mother who has Alzheimer's disease too.

We all begin as caregivers with the best of intentions but soon discover that cleaning portable toilets and changing adult diapers can be less than uplifting. Holding someone in your arms as he or she dies is not fun. Still, it's possible that the quality of life remaining for your loved ones, and for yourself in the midst of giving care, can be lightened, heightened, and brightened simply by your approach to it. We just have to remember to laugh.

Now my wife is battling breast cancer. She was diagnosed as Stage Two and lost a breast, several lymph nodes, and nearly her sense of humor. Today she is successfully confronting her disease and beating it by not granting it any strength through fear. She has pursued all the accepted medical cures, from a radical mastectomy to two protocols of chemotherapy stacked one after the other. She is additionally following an Aryuvedic doctor's regimen and a healthy diet. She exercises, eats just enough chocolate to keep her soul healthy, and laughs often. Her prognosis is good because her quality of life is as high as her spirits, regardless of the cancer (some days, she says, because of the cancer).

Learn to laugh. Above all, learn how to help others laugh. Don't be afraid of looking ridiculous; seek it. Don't be afraid others will be offended by black humor; force it upon them. Shove it down their throats until they gag and spew it out their noses, just as we did as kids when we laughed too hard with our milk and cookies. There are no time-outs in warm kitchens with Moms baking cookies for cancer patients, no retreat from the school-yard bully when the bully follows you home, right up to your bedroom, sleeps with you, and beats you up from the inside. The only way to defeat a bully is not to fear him. We all know that. What we forget when we fear too much is that the only way to defeat fear is to laugh.

This book is billed as a survival manual for the caregiver. I hope it's really a pebble dropped into a pond. Everyone follows another's example, but examples have to start somewhere. Be a ripple; pass it on. Create other ripples.

Never forget: Cancer is not contagious. Laughter is.

Exercises for Chapter One

Rent a funny video.

Make popcorn.

Buy a joke-a-day calendar.

Play a prank on your patient.

Laugh at yourself every day.

Chapter Two

Where to Begin, or Is It Beguine?

In 1935, Cole Porter wrote a song he called "Begin the Beguine" for a musical on Broadway called *Jubilee*. Although the Beguine is technically a native dance of Martinique and St. Lucia, we opportunistic Americans adopted it and made it into a ballroom dance similar to the rumba. To the natives of Martinique, the Beguine is the dance of life, a dance filled with the rhythms of exuberance and romance.

Every dance begins with the first step. Of course, dancing really starts even before you hear the music. I know some very fortunate people who can even dance without any music. I consider them truly remarkable, though I don't think they're any more courageous or flamboyant than the rest of us. I think to dance without music is something any of us can do. Just as with anything else, you simply have to start. Put one foot out, then the other, and suddenly you're dancing.

So it is with the dance of life. You begin with just one step. Don't worry about the second or third, where your hands are supposed to be, or when you'll twirl your partner. The dips and twirls will take care of themselves.

In December of 1996, Marthy, my partner in the dance, traveled with me all the way to Oregon to be supportive as I underwent surgery to remove a cyst from my pancreas. We left our cottage while dodging fallen trees between blizzards—leaving Vashon Island, Washington, on the tail of one storm and arriving in Oregon in the teeth of another.

We checked into a motel in Newberg. We expected to be absent a week, the week my surgeon had told me I'd spend in the hospital recuperating. We planned to stay one night in the motel waiting out the storm, waiting for the morning when I'd be admitted to the hospital. That morning, Marthy discovered a lump in her left breast. She didn't say a word about it. She walked me through the snowdrifts to the hospital and kissed me for good luck as they wheeled me into surgery.

When my surgeon, Dr. Covey, found her in the lobby to assure her that the operation had gone as expected, she calmly asked him for a referral for a mammogram. She'd inquired that morning at the radiology department but had been told she needed a referral from her doctor and that the soonest appointment available was a week later. She was in a strange city with her regular doctor two hundred miles away.

Dr. Covey listened to her request, then walked out of the room. He returned a few minutes later.

"Go on back; they're waiting for you," he said.

She told me about the lump when I arrived in my room from Recovery an hour later.

We were stunned. The immediacy of my condition was too recent; we were barely beyond escaping it and just beginning to breathe easier. Now, Marthy had breast cancer. It wasn't fair; they had to be wrong. We'd wait for the results of the mammogram, not waste energy worrying about something that probably wasn't even real. We hugged as much as the surgery on my stomach would allow.

Dr. Covey met with Marthy on his break from surgery for lunch. The lump was suspicious, he said. It had to come out.

We remained stunned. I remember feeling numb. We maintained our stoic wait-and-see approach. We told ourselves that "suspicious" didn't have to mean cancer. We reassured each other in my hospital room, telling lies until we began to believe them.

"No way," we said to each other. "It's like my pancreas—not malignant. Nothing to worry about; it's a false alarm. We've got too much to do."

I remember Marthy said, "At least I've got great veins if I have to take chemo."

Dr. Covey took Marthy's lump the next day. The nurses commented on what great veins she had—so easy for them to find for the IVs. For three days we hung out in my hospital room waiting for the pathology report. For three days we told each other the same lies, over and over again. We believed them more with every telling. Marthy walked me around the ward, helping me get my legs back, getting ready to go home.

On Friday, Dr. Covey told Marthy the lump was malignant and that he hadn't taken as much tissue as he needed to remove. There was to be more surgery for her, a partial mastectomy. He scheduled it for the beginning of the following week. Saturday morning he released me from the hospital two days early.

"Go home and take care of your lady," he said and then amended himself. "Or go back to your motel, I should say."

He laughed.

"How long have you been there now?" he asked.

"Six days," I said.

I suppose he intended us to occupy ourselves with activities that might take our minds off the impending repeat surgery for Marthy. My digestive track was so virginal following my surgery that I didn't dare become acquainted with any environs greater than ten feet from an available, functioning toilet. We discovered our motel provided us with several premium cable-movie channels. We spent the weekend in our queen-size bed watching television and listening to the snow melt and lying to each other.

"I'm not worried," we said to one another.

"If you've got to have cancer, this is the best one to have," we said.

They took a third of Marthy's left breast on Monday and eighteen lymph nodes from her left armpit. They also installed a couple of small plastic balls, reservoirs into which the liquids of her wounds would drain for the next week. These globes hung from tubes along her side, stretching nearly to her waist. She pinned them to her blouses to keep them from flopping about. I joked that she could hold them under her arm and when she wanted to fill out her cleavage a little, flap her arm to pump her breast up. Whenever she stood, she began to clasp her left hand in her right, close to her chest. I called it her Jack Benny phase. Whenever she'd strike the pose waiting for elevators or lost in the aisles of the Newberg Fred Meyer, I'd call out, "Oh, Rochester." Sometimes it made her laugh.

Wednesday the tests came back.

"Your cancer is intraductile," Dr. Covey told Marthy. "The rest of the ducts are about to erupt. We have to take the whole breast off. You have vascular involvement as well. The good news is that only three of your lymph nodes were involved. Your cancer is in stage two, not three."

They scheduled her third surgery for the following Friday. For two days we lay around our motel room. Our primary sources of distraction were watching movies on HBO and me going to and from the bathroom. And lying to each other.

"I'm still not scared," we said to each other.

"Stage two is much better than stage three," we said.

That Friday they took the rest of Marthy's left breast. She was so frightened by her third surgery in as many weeks that her great veins shriveled and disappeared. We didn't know where they went and the nurses couldn't tell us. They were no longer to be found in her arms. One of her favorite nurses, and by this time she'd been around the Newberg Hospital long enough to have developed favorites, was unable to start the IV. After several attempts, the nurse suggested that Marthy wait and let the anesthesiologist begin the IV in surgery. Marthy requested that they wait until after she'd been sedated. It must have worked because she didn't have an IV when they wheeled her through the double doors of the prep room that morning, but she did when she emerged several hours later. We didn't ask if they had had any difficulty starting it. Sometimes it's better to let experts do their jobs behind closed doors.

Marthy remained in the hospital for a few days following her surgery and then returned to our motel room. I was weak, without stamina, and needed to nap frequently during the day. She was cranked up and unable to sit still. I helped bathe her, held her when she cried, and listened when she needed to be angry and vent her fears. She urged me to eat and helped find solutions to my dehydration.

Trapped in a small, rented room, we discovered we had become each other's caregivers. Maybe that's what's really going on whenever any of us give care to another. We do it as much for ourselves as we do it for our loved ones. Maybe that's why our loved ones allow us to care for them: they realize we need to do something to contribute, or else we'd go crazy from sitting around and feeling helpless. Whichever it is, the chicken or the egg, it's a symbiotic relationship between caregiver and patient—one that benefits both.

So I made jokes about Jack Benny and inflatable boobs. Marthy made jokes about the frequency and length of my trips to the bathroom. I called her Booby; she called me Poopy. The motel and hospital staff called us by our first names. Friends and relatives dropped in as if we'd moved to a new home. We checked in for one night and checked out thirty days later.

There you have it: our beginning, which has meant the end of anything that might have approached "normal" in our lives. Our story is a good one—rich with pathos and comedy. As hard as it's been, we're emerging wiser and happier for having experienced it. You have a beginning also, a story every bit as rich as ours. It began when your regular existence ended, when your loved one was initially diagnosed with cancer.

Think about your own story. Write it down, even if only in an outline form. Remind yourself of how it began, of that moment when everything remained the same but would never be the same again. Accept that it's happened, and you can respond to it. Remember: Every ending is a beginning; it can be the start of something good or of something bad. It's up to you. Don't be afraid to learn to dance. The dips and twirls will take care of themselves.

EXERCISES FOR CHAPTER TWO

Learn a new dance step.

Waltz your partner around the kitchen.

Whistle a tune no matter how badly.

Chapter Three

Buying a Ticket to Ride, or It Helps If You Scream on the Way Down

An issue of *Reader's Digest* that I found in our surgeon's office in Newberg quoted comic Jerry Seinfeld as saying he thinks life is like a roller coaster: at the end, the most we can hope for is that we haven't thrown up and our hair isn't mussed. Though he made me laugh, I don't believe Mr. Seinfeld has ever been a chemo patient.

Chemotherapy patients have no fear of losing their cookies. They accept vomiting as part of their diet. Chemo patients also have no fear of mussing their hair. They do wonder, however, just what kind of hair they'll have to muss when it finally begins to grow back. They know, from the experience of others, that it won't be the same as it was before they had chemotherapy; but then, neither will they. Cancer and chemo change people, both patients and caregivers.

Prepare for the roller coaster of chemotherapy. It won't do you any good, but it will give you a false sense of security. As long as you don't punish yourself once you discover just how un-ready you really are, it won't hurt you to begin without fear. If you're a patient, expect your emotions to run the full gamut while your body runs the full gauntlet of depletion by overt toxicity. If you're a caregiver, be prepared for anything, and be flexible.

Chemotherapy is poison. It's supposed to stop all reproduction of cells. If you consider the fact that when people die their cells continue to reproduce, which makes their hair and nails continue to grow, you will begin to understand why your patient feels like he or she is dying. It's because he or she is dying. Nails stop growing. Hair falls out. Your patient is walking around in a body that stopped living just after the second treatment. Living inside a dead body can shatter emotions and send humor for a walk on the gallows side. Suddenly, the smallest advance becomes a delight, while the most trivial setback triggers deep depression.

Just as with any roller coaster ride, it really does help to scream all the way down. As it does when lifting weights or giving birth, exhaling helps lessen the pain during cancer treatment. Sometimes when the pain isn't physical, the need to scream becomes even greater.

When I need to scream, I go into the woods that surround our little cottage and scream at the Universe. I don't believe the Universe hears me, much less listens, but I feel better for having expressed myself.

Marthy doesn't scream. I've tried to help her, but this is an area where caregivers must tread lightly. Trying to help a patient vent anger at the Universe often results in a scream, but not one directed at anything quite so ephemeral as the Cosmos.

"I can't scream," Marthy said when I suggested she step into the trees and release her frustrations.

"You're a woman," I observed. "Can't all women scream?"

"Very funny," she said.

I hadn't intended to be funny.

"I'm quite serious," I said. "Women are always screaming in the movies."

"You want to hear screaming?" Marthy said, her voice rising.

"Not particularly," I answered and headed for the computer room.

"And what do you know about women?" she said following me. "You didn't even notice when your ex-girlfriend cut me up at that birthday party."

"Birthday party?"

28

"The one in Portland I didn't want to go to, the one you insisted we attend," she said, her voice another octave higher.

"That was over a year ago," I said.

"That's the point. It still hurts and you still don't care," she said, her eyes brimming, her voice shaking.

"I do care. I just didn't see it happen, that's all."

"And now you diminish it just because you didn't see it happen. You think I made it all up."

"I didn't say that, sweetie. I said I didn't see it happen."

"I don't want to live this way," she said shrilly. "I'm leaving."

She didn't leave, of course, but maybe I should have. I should have gone out into the woods myself instead of trying to make her do so. Sometimes, a caregiver shouldn't try to help but should sit back and watch. We caregivers need to learn when to keep our mouths shut and listen instead.

Listening is truly the key to being a great conversationalist. Listening is also key to being a good partner and caregiver. I guess the trick to the "screaming thing" is to stay focused on who or what one should be screaming at. Sometimes it's the Universe. Sometimes it's the caregiver. Sometimes it's the doctor, a friend, or even the patient. There's simply something about cancer and fear that needs yelling about. You'll get yelled at too. Sometimes you'll deserve it, and sometimes you won't. Remember that deserving the blame isn't what it's all about: yelling is.

EXERCISES FOR CHAPTER THREE

Find someplace quiet and scream at the top of your lungs.

Take your patient someplace quiet where he or she can scream as
loud as possible.

Don't scream in a public place unless you can afford a fine for
disturbing the peace.

Chapter Four

Eating the Elephant

When your patient is first facing months of chemotherapy, the task may seem insurmountable. Remind your patient that each journey begins with a single step. Remember to focus on the first step only, not the end of the trip. If we look too far ahead, we can lose sight of the immediate, take a wrong turn, or worse, step into a pothole.

Recently, when I was intimidated by the size of a large project, a friend reminded me that the only way to eat an elephant is one bite at a time. If you look at the entire elephant before you begin the meal, you might lose your appetite. It occurs to me that elephants are similar to chemotherapy in that both look better from a little ways off, rather than up close and personal. And finding yourself facing either may not be much fun.

Most chemotherapy regimens call for six months or less in treatment. Marthy underwent six months of regular chemotherapy, if there is such a thing, and then five months of Taxol treatment immediately thereafter. Eleven months of consistent chemotherapy is a long time to suffer, but she was indomitable throughout, rarely complaining although she suffered the same nausea, hair loss, fatigue, and aches and pains as most other patients. With the Taxol, she suffered severe neuropathy as well, which resulted in permanent nerve damage to her hands, feet, and eyes.

When she had completed the treatments, I asked her what had helped her the most to get through them.

"The bright spot you gave me every day," she said. "Every day, you helped me find something beautiful, or funny, or tender. That, and having my new granddaughter, Madison, with me. Her innocence helped me see the best in life."

Marthy's comments regarding her granddaughter came as no surprise. Simply being with Madison had proved enough to lift her spirits, regardless of how difficult the time. But I was surprised by her comments regarding the bright spots.

I hadn't realized I was finding something bright to show Marthy every day. I'd just been trying to help her live normally, as she'd requested when she first began chemotherapy. Looking back now, I see the greatest gift caregivers can offer chemo patients may be to do just that: help them live as normal a life as possible.

Try to continue life together as if there were no chemical interruptions. When the side effects of chemotherapy intervene, work around them without making too big a deal about the inconvenience. We're all inconvenienced by something every day. If we labor and lament over inconveniences, we lessen the quality of our lives, with or without chemo. Finding happiness while in chemotherapy depends on something as simple as always looking on the bright side, just as it does in our normal lives.

Point out the beauty in a sunrise or sunset, the peace of a starlit night, the calming sound of rain drumming on your roof. Seek humor in all that happens, especially the unpleasant things. If you have children, spend happy times with them. Marthy's granddaughter could make her laugh with a cockeyed grin, a hiccup, or even a filled diaper. Look for the beauty to share with your patient and you'll discover a lift in your own spirits as well.

I romanced my Marthy at the times when she felt the most unattractive. I brought her flowers when there was no occasion to celebrate. I danced her around the house to silly songs I made up about breasts and nausea and what she calls "chemo-brain." We found ways to make her trips to the clinic for chemotherapy more fun. I drove her past pretty views of the city or along the waterfront. When she had to lie down to rest, I often lay with her and held her. When she was tired but couldn't sleep, I sang her lullabies. Instead of helping her rest, my voice made her laugh.

Find something to treat yourselves to each time you take your patient for a treatment. Find something pleasant to anticipate each time your patient must see the doctor. Look for the good news around you and surround your patient with ideas that lift up rather than weigh down.

Get a calendar and mark off the treatments as they pass so your patient can see the progress made. Help your patient realize that as the treatments progress, he or she will naturally feel worse. Remind your patient that feeling worse as he or she gets better is all part of the twisted plan that is chemotherapy.

Read the chapter titled "Looking for Four-Leaf Clovers, or Pebbling the Walk." Find a project you can accomplish concurrently with the schedule of chemotherapy. As the project nears completion, the patient will be reminded that the chemotherapy regimen nears its end also. Jigsaw puzzles are popular because they don't take up much space or energy. Collecting pretty stones off the beach or flowers to dry for an arrangement can excite your patient's senses just when the nuts and bolts of living seem to be the hardest to handle.

You, the caregiver, must provide the spice that makes each bite of the elephant appealing. You know your patient better than anyone. Be a creative chef.

EXERCISES FOR CHAPTER FOUR

Sing in the shower loud enough for your patient to hear you.

Start a project together.

Buy a calendar and mark off the treatments.

Bring little presents home.

Chapter Five

Hollow Victories, Solid Defeats

There are times in our lives when losing is the only way we can win. Sometimes when the bully is much bigger than we are, it's simply wiser to curl up on the saloon floor, protect our vital organs, and take our licking. My generation learned this from Maverick. Maverick never stood up to a bully who was very much bigger or faster on the draw if he could help it. He taught us a wise person is sometimes the one who runs away and lives to run another day.

This is contradictory to the Gary Cooper/Jimmy Stewart ethic, however. Those guys never ran, no matter which movie you picked. They demanded that we all stand up for what we believe no matter what the odds. But have you ever known someone who actually did this? Think about it. Those who actually stood up to forces beyond their measure are hard to remember, probably because being run over by a freight train while denying that a train is approaching proves hazardous to your health.

I remember a poem about John Brown, the abolitionist, I read as a child. I can't remember its exact words, but I will never forget its message: even though John Brown was right, he was killed just the same, as if he'd been wrong.

I suspect Mr. Brown stood up to the forces of slavery not because he expected to win or even to survive, but to set an example. Whatever John Brown did or didn't expect, he stood in front of a fast moving train and then lay smolderin' in the grave. The example he set has lasted for generations and still stands today for people of all colors, but if you aren't intending to set an example that will lead an entire people to freedom, duck when the cancer hammer comes around.

Help your patient reserve his or her energies for fights that can be won, not empty gestures. Don't expect fair play. Your patient is facing the biggest, scariest bully of them all and pitting another bully, nearly as big and scary, against it. This becomes an odd dance where we resist one by not resisting the other. Taking chemo is a choice, the choice of life. This is a bully you should not run from, should not strike back at, and should not resist in any way.

Marthy and I have friends who are deeply involved with alternative healing practices. These friends were initially appalled by the side effects of Marthy's chemotherapy and offered solutions to the discomfort and nausea she experienced. At first we were receptive to their remedies, but soon realized that, upon closer examination, the remedies often conflicted with the intended effect of the chemotherapy. Though we cleared everything through Marthy's oncologist, he often didn't know about the effects of the herbs and other natural medications. He simply waved them through his checkpoint.

Our personal research revealed that certain herbs are antioxidants and would work to flush the toxins out of Marthy—the very toxins designed to suppress all rapid cell regeneration and kill the cancer. In other words, taking antioxidants while taking toxicants is like pushing and pulling at the same time. One would defeat the other, even if only in a stalemate. Marthy had to accept the poisoning of the chemotherapy, because that's what it is supposed to do: poison the patient.

So what can you do to help your patient? Accept what you can and cannot do to effect a return to health. Help yourself to understand that when your patient feels lousy, it's good news. When your patient is throwing up the dinner you so carefully planned and executed, it's more good news. The chemo is working. You begin to realize that in the topsy-turvy world of cancer and chemotherapy, what used to be good can now be bad, and what used to be bad can now either be good or bad.

Sounds crazy, but in the world of chemotherapy, sometimes up is down, and sometimes down is up. Remember that sometimes throwing up and feeling down is really on the way up, not on the way down.

EXERCISES FOR CHAPTER FIVE

Laugh out loud in a public place and watch the faces around you.

Lie on your back and imagine the world upside down.

Pick a fight with the universe using your pillow as a stand-in.

Chapter Six

Be an Advocate, Not an Avocado

You must be aware of more than your own concern while you're a caregiver for a chemo patient. Whether or not your patient asks you to be, you must become an advocate. Attend all meetings with your patient's doctors, pay attention to all discussions, and take notes regarding all possible treatments, as well as the ones your patient is receiving. Don't sit quietly like a vegetable. If you hear something you don't understand, speak up. If you see something you don't like, say so. Ask questions, get answers, and become involved.

No matter how many times we hear things, each time we hear them, we hear them differently. Each of us hears everything differently than another can. A patient whose body and mind are being buffeted by chemotherapy cannot be expected to remember all of the many details necessary to keep treatment appointments and medications in concert. Neither can a caregiver, who is watching a loved one suffer, be expected to keep everything straight. Stress scatters your attention no matter how good your intention to keep things straight. Staying on top of the myriad details involved with chemotherapy will take both of you.

Marthy and I would commonly emerge from her oncologist's office with entirely different memories of what he'd discussed with us. Dr. Goodman was extremely conscientious in his explanations of treatments, options, conditions, and expectations; yet, no matter how carefully he spoke, Marthy and I would come away with differing accounts of the visit. At first the differences in our versions disturbed us; neither was ever entirely correct, and it worried us that we couldn't be more competent. Gradually we realized that hearing things differently wasn't important. What was important was that we were both trying and that by disagreeing, we were able to sort the information out between us. Whenever we disagreed on something, we were careful to ask for clarification and so were much more thorough than either of us might have been working alone.

Prior to the onset of her Taxol treatments, Dr. Goodman was careful to explain what symptoms and side effects Marthy should expect. Among them was a tingling and numbness in her extremities—usually fingers and toes. Knowing Marthy to be stoic regarding her discomfort during her first six months of chemotherapy, he cautioned her to be forthcoming regarding everything she experienced. He stressed the importance of open communication between doctor and patient. She agreed, and I made a mental note to observe her even more closely.

She began to experience a tingling in her fingertips and toes immediately following her first Taxol treatment and dutifully reported those sensations to Dr. Goodman at her next appointment.

"Don't be concerned," he reassured her. "Remember that I told you this would probably happen. It's a normal side effect of the Taxol."

With the second treatment, the tingling progressed to a light numbness. She again reported the sensations, as well as other symptoms she was experiencing. Again he reassured her.

The numbness continued to progress through the third treatment. She reported to him at the following appointment and was again reassured. This cycle continued until she was ready for the final treatment early in December. She'd been preparing herself for this last treatment, checking the schedule and hoping she'd be sufficiently recovered in time to enjoy Christmas. The numbness had continued to progress, until she likened the sensation in her hands to that of wearing thick mittens. She was unable to knit or to open jars or even to perform a multitude of lesser manipulative tasks. Her feet had become so numb that she could walk barefoot on cold linoleum without complaint. Her eyes no longer focused sufficiently to allow her to read. We worried, but when you're fighting cancer, worrying is not unusual. We believed the symptoms would reverse themselves. The doctor had told us so.

"This is normal," we said to each other. "Normal for Taxol treatments, that is."

A couple of days before her last appointment, I came home to find her rocking in her chair, holding herself and whimpering.

"What's wrong?" I asked.

"I fell off the porch today," she said.

I examined her injuries. Her arm and leg on one side were turning black and purple.

"How'd you fall off the porch?" I asked.

"I don't know," she said. "I just turned around and suddenly I was falling. I guess I stepped off the edge."

She laughed at herself. A couple of years before, she'd fallen off a bulkhead at the beach while pulling blackberry vines.

"I guess I've done it again," she said, referring to her blackberry bruises.

When we saw Dr. Goodman a couple of days later, she mentioned the fall to him. He examined her bruises with concern.

"Tell me again how you did this?" he asked.

Marthy explained again, adding, "Maybe my numb feet didn't help. I couldn't tell if my foot was on the porch when I stepped."

"Your feet are numb?" he asked with surprise.

"Well, yes," Marthy answered, "you said it was a normal side effect of the Taxol."

"I said tingling and numbness in the fingertips and toes," he said with concern. "Show me how much is numb."

Marthy pointed up to her ankles and then up to her wrists. She told him about her failing eyesight.

"Just how bad is your vision?" he asked.

"I can't read anymore unless it's really large print," Marthy told him.

"I'll be back in just a bit," Dr. Goodman said. He left the room. He returned in a few minutes.

He had tears in his eyes. I felt a cold lump in the pit of my stomach.

"I've got good news and bad news," he said.

"Tell me the good news," Marthy said slowly.

"We're not going to give you another dose of Taxol today. You're all done," he said.

"That's not good news," Marthy said. "Tell me the bad news."

The tears returned to his eyes.

"We may have gone too far already," he said. "Sometimes, if it's too extensive, the nerve damage is irreversible."

"My feeling may not come back?" Marthy asked.

"Your feeling may not come back," Dr. Goodman nodded. "And sometimes the nerves continue to deteriorate even after the treatment has stopped. Your nerve damage may continue to worsen."

Marthy cried a little.

"I'm sorry," he said, crying a little also. "You were supposed to tell me what was happening as the treatments progressed. We would have stopped the treatments if we'd known."

"I thought I was telling you," Marthy said. "I thought the numbness was supposed to progress with the treatments; all the other symptoms got worse as the treatments went on."

We talked about what had gone wrong and realized that at each visit, all Marthy had told Dr. Goodman was that the tingling and numbness continued. While she meant the symptoms had continued to progress, he understood her to mean they had continued to the same degree.

"All we can do now is wait," Dr. Goodman said.

So we waited. Marthy was lucky. Months later, most of her nerves regenerated. She can read and knit again, but still suffers residual numbness in her hands and feet. She doesn't talk about it much, but I watched her take a steaming basket out of a pan of boiling water the other night with her bare fingers. She never flinched.

No matter how carefully you think you've listened to every detail, double-check everything. Re-state what you understand, and ask for corroboration. We can't face what we don't know. It's always the miscommunications or non-communications that ultimately come back to harm us.

Sometimes, some of us are unable to follow the complex details that chemotherapy entails. If you can't be an advocate, don't pretend to be one. Work within your strengths, and don't be embarrassed to admit when you discover a weakness in yourself. Remember that this is not about you or your pride. You are not in a contest to see who can be the best caregiver. Instead, you are contesting for your loved one's life.

If you find the medical details overwhelming, ask someone else to fulfill that role for your patient. Never expect the patient to deal with all the details by him or herself. Chemotherapy scrambles the mind at times so that a patient cannot always perform a task adequately. "What will I blame it on after the therapy is over?" she asked one night after she'd done something silly.

"What did you blame it on before chemotherapy?" I asked.

Looking back now, I feel responsible for the miscommunication with Dr. Goodman. Marthy, of course, blames herself. We all blame ourselves and no one else. It remains to this day a hard lesson learned: no matter how careful we are, misunderstandings still occur.

Do your best, but don't expect to be perfect. Don't be afraid to ask for help when you need it. Don't sit by like a vegetable expecting everyone else to take care of the details.

Anyone can get an avocado at a supermarket. Advocates are not purchased by the pound. Advocates grow only out of love and stand up for their loved ones when they cannot stand up for themselves. Pay attention and speak up when necessary. Be an advocate, not an avocado.

EXERCISES FOR CHAPTER SIX

Post a list of your patient's medications.

Post a calendar with your patient's appointments.

Keep a notebook handy for questions to ask the doctor.

Buy a few avocados and make guacamole.

Chapter Seven

Feeding Time at the Zoo

No manual for caregivers would be complete without a chapter on the care and feeding of your patient. Unlike other members of the animal kingdom, chemotherapy patients cannot be trained to eat at specific times of the day. Their appetites will not fit conveniently into your schedule, nor will their tastes always match your menu. Feeding times at the chemotherapy zoo will be at the patient's discretion or not at all.

My brother Christopher was easy to care for but impossible to feed. No matter what tempted his palate, it never stayed down. Before long, anything he found appetizing also nauseated him. His favorite dishes lost their attraction forever.

Once, a couple close to Chris invited us to their house for dinner. They prepared a meal they knew to be among his favorites: a casserole of chicken, cheese, and broccoli. Much to his embarrassment and their chagrin, he managed to swallow only a small portion before he became violently ill. He rushed from the table and barely beat his dinner to the bathroom, leaving me to continue polite conversation with his friends. From that night on, he couldn't stomach even the thought of that casserole. During the several courses of chemotherapy he underwent in the next five years, he was forced to develop entirely new tastes in food. So completely had he exhausted his options, that by the time he died, his tastes had come nearly full circle. He never did, however, develop a taste for Brussels sprouts.

Chemotherapy protocols have progressed leaps and bounds since Chris underwent treatment. The degree of nausea he experienced is unusual today. My sister Karen underwent similar treatment just four years later and actually gained weight during her chemotherapy. She still experienced nausea, but whatever appetite stimulant her doctor prescribed worked so well that she ate in spite of her queasiness. However encouraging, Karen's experience can't be expected. Patients must be compelled to eat regularly, because the introduction of toxins into a person's system can steal an appetite more rapidly than any flu.

Prompting Marthy to eat regularly proved to be an ongoing ordeal. At first I carefully planned menus I knew to be her favorites, but when the meal was ready, Marthy was rarely interested. I soon discovered that if she said she felt like eating rice, I'd better get a bowl in front of her within ten minutes or forget it entirely. Waiting until dinnertime to offer what she'd wanted that afternoon was an exercise in futility.

I stocked the pantry with odds and ends rather than preplanned menu-items so that I'd be ready to throw together whatever she might find attractive at a moment's notice. If she said she felt like corn or another fresh vegetable I couldn't stock on a regular basis, I'd rush to the market to get it, rush home to fix it, and put it in front of her no matter what the time of day. When it comes to feeding a chemotherapy patient, haste does not make waste.

At first we tried to stick to a healthy regimen, but after a while just getting anything into her took priority over what kind of food it might be. If we were driving through the city and she suddenly had a craving for a cheeseburger, we stopped and found a cheeseburger. I, of course, ate with her whenever she felt the urge. I, of course, gained weight while she continued to lose it. She, at times, suffered mild nausea; I often suffered severe indigestion. I learned to travel with a pocketful of antacids. I still do.

For general nausea, we found my Grandmother Reed's remedy for upset stomach useful. Grate an apple from which you've pared the skin.

The fruit is easy to digest in grated form and replaces fluids with its juice, and the pectin helps to slow the patient's system in both directions.

For severe diarrhea, Grandma's remedy is steamed, skinless potato eaten dry without seasoning. I'm sure your family has its own remedies. Don't be afraid to try them. Believing a cure will work is often the reason it does.

When Marthy began Taxol therapy, her irregular eating reversed itself. She used to go long periods without meals; after Taxol, she wanted to eat all of the time. During one three-hour Taxol infusion treatment, I watched her consume a large vegetarian sandwich, a large tuna-salad sandwich, a bowl of soup, three cookies the size of dessert plates, and two cans of soda. Although the volume of her intake increased dramatically during the Taxol treatments, her tastes remained specific and eccentric.

For instance, Marthy developed a craving for the top crusts of chocolate covered old-fashioned cake donuts from a specific bakery, but only the top crusts. Or deep-fried halibut pieces, without chips, from a local seafood restaurant. Or a cheeseburger from a specific fast-food chain. She never ate these kinds of food before she was diagnosed with cancer. This diet seemed to come about as a result of the chemotherapy, the Taxol in particular.

One of Marthy's cravings has remained constant before, during, and after chemotherapy. She loves Jell-O, particularly cherry Jell-O. I've never seen anyone enjoy a bowl of Jell-O as much as Marthy. We still keep a bowl of Jell-O in the fridge at all times.

Prepare to be unprepared when it comes to feeding your patient. Don't expect him or her to want to eat whatever you've labored to prepare. Expect to be as spontaneous as his or her gustatory whims in order to keep your patient eating regularly.

Pay attention. If your patient says he or she craves a particular food or dish, don't argue. Don't parent your loved one with reminders of calories or fat content. Fix what he or she wants, or go get it. Do whatever you have to do; the important thing is to keep your patient eating.

The key to feeding chemotherapy patients is to remember that in order to keep a vehicle operating, you have to fuel it. We'd all like to put only premium fuel in our vehicles, but we have to face the fact that sometimes we have to settle for the lower-grade stuff. You can worry about returning to a healthy diet once the chemotherapy is over. So chew on that for a while. See if you can get your patient to chew on it as well.

EXERCISES FOR CHAPTER SEVEN

Make a list of your patient's favorite foods.

Stock up on the favorites.

Fix your patient a snack right now.

Watch your own weight as well as your patient's.

Chapter Eight
Two Heads Are Better Than One

Three weeks after Marthy started chemotherapy, her hair began falling out just as her doctor had advised her it probably would. She called me into the bathroom and pointed at the hair in the tub. She laughed and said she guessed she wasn't going to be one of the lucky few who didn't lose their hair during treatment.

I asked if she was frightened by the prospect of going bald.

"No," she said, "I should have expected it." But then her tears began and she moved into my arms.

I remember when my little brother Chris lost his hair during his initial round of chemotherapy. He awoke one morning to find clumps on his pillow. He said it so disconcerted him that he shaved his head immediately rather than face another morning like that. He said seeing his hair on the pillow and then plucking fingers-full from his head was the most graphic reminder of his body's demise he'd ever experienced.

Hair is an icon of vanity in our culture. Male baldness, and the avoidance of it, is the bait that fishes several million dollars a year from our social pond. I've seen surveys in which women claim they find a bald man equally as attractive as a man with a full head of hair. I've also seen polls that indicate that when women are offered five men to date with all other factors equal, ladies will choose a man with hair over one without. I haven't read any polls in which men were asked if they preferred bald women.

Men have come to expect a degree of hair loss as they age. Women have not. When men shave their heads, people may assume they do so out of vanity. No one assumes vanity is the motive when they see a bald woman.

When Marthy's hair began to fall out, I told her that when she shaved her head, I'd shave mine too.

"You don't have to do that," she said, but her eyes were already laughing at the thought.

I knew when I looked at her that once I'd offered, I had to follow through.

She called Jim, her hair stylist, for an appointment and made two, one for each of us. When the day came, we arrived to find Jim's shop closed to all but us. He didn't want Marthy to suffer from an audience.

Jim's wife, Charlene, watched with me as Jim shaved Marthy's head; then Marthy and Charlene watched him shave mine. When Jim was through, he produced a small camera, and Charlene snapped a shot of him standing between Marthy and myself. My severed ponytail dangled from one of his hands like a trophy trout.

I asked him what we owed him.

"No charge," he said. "It's the least I can do."

We walked out of Jim's shop feeling nude. A couple of strangers, headed into Earl's hardware store, stopped, and smiled at us. On the way to our car, a child pointed and tugged on his mother's arm. It was our first exposure to the kind of attention we would draw for the next eleven months. Marthy covered her head with her hands once she was safely inside the car.

"Take me to the grocery store," she said, "before I chicken out."

Marthy's son Todd worked in a local supermarket. When she'd told him she would be losing her hair, he'd said he didn't want to see his mother bald. She knew he'd been kidding, but she also understood the edge beneath the tease. He was uncertain of his own reaction and didn't want to hurt her.

"I have to get this over with," Marthy said. "I've got to see Todd."

I parked in front of the store and asked if she wanted me to go in with her.

"No," she said. "This is something I need to do alone."

Ten minutes later she was back in the car, her face in her lap. I couldn't tell if she was laughing or crying.

"Are you laughing or crying?" I asked.

"A little of both," she said and sat up.

"How'd it go?" I asked.

"Todd backed away, and kept saying, 'Oh shit!' But he was laughing. It was okay," she said.

She looked at me thoughtfully.

"Everyone in there stared at me," she said. "And then I realized that people don't wear wigs for their own comfort. They wear them for everyone else's."

"Do you want to buy a wig?" I asked.

"Nope," she said. She ran a hand over her smooth scalp. "This is for me. If you can go bald, so can I."

So we did, for eleven months. Marthy often wore a hat, especially when she felt cold, but for the most part we went hatless. People stared. Sometimes people were rude, but most of the time strangers were sympathetic and often came forward to reveal they too had survived cancer and chemotherapy.

We discovered that people in the Seattle area, with its many cancer treatment and research centers, treated us with respect and sometimes deference. When we traveled in Oregon, people appeared to be less understanding. Once we stopped at a small donut store just outside Newport on the Oregon coast. The shop was known for its German potato donuts and had been a favorite stopping spot for my family on camping trips when I was a child.

I was surprised and pleased to find the original owner still operating the store. Now in his eighties, he peered at us through thick spectacles as we perused his pastries. He was not the warm and engaging proprietor I remembered from my childhood. He stayed back from the counter and only looked in our direction occasionally, as though frightened of us in some way. Finally, after we'd made our selections and he was sacking them for us, he looked directly at us.

"Do you mind if I ask you a personal question?" he asked in a thick accent (without smiling).

"Not at all," we said.

"Are you members of some kind of sect or something?" he asked.

We laughed, and Marthy explained to him her situation.

"Ah," he said and smiled broadly. "My wife is not doing so well either. We may have to close the store after all these years."

And then the friendly proprietor I recalled from my youth emerged, and we commiserated in the way only comrades of a common cause can.

After that encounter, whenever someone asked us if we belonged to a sect, I would answer, "Yes. We're heterosexuals."

As common as cancers and chemotherapy are today, many people still asked thoughtless questions. One man stared at Marthy for several minutes in a drugstore while they were both waiting for prescriptions. Finally he approached her and pointed to her head.

"How long did you have to think about that before you did it?" he asked.

She explained her chemotherapy and then spent the next fifteen minutes consoling him for having asked such an insensitive question.

A stranger approached me on the ferry to Vashon Island one day. "I didn't think much of you before," he said, pumping my hand. "But since you shaved your head for your wife, you've elevated yourself in my book. Buddy, you're all right!" I still don't know this individual, but he waves at me whenever our cars pass on the highway.

Another stranger approached me in the supermarket on a different day. He wasn't smiling. "I hope you realize you've made all the rest of us husbands look bad," he said. This man does not wave at me.

Several women approached both Marthy and myself on many occasions to tell us what a wonderful example Marthy set with her courage to walk about in public without covering her head, without hiding her cancer, displaying her undiminished humor and love of life for all to see. We, of course, did not shave our heads for any of the people who derived either pleasure or displeasure from our display. We did it for ourselves.

I thought I shaved my head just for Marthy, to remind her that no matter how difficult her treatment might become, she was never facing it alone. If people suggested that I shaved my head in sympathy, I would correct them. "I like to call it a solidarity shave," I'd say.

Though shaving our heads together reassured Marthy just as I'd hoped, what I gained was quite different and unexpected: I was suddenly a hero. Not to any adoring public, but to Marthy. Marthy thought I was a champion for having the courage to shave my head for her. As a result, I began to think of myself as a hero too. Somehow, seeing myself as a hero made doing heroic deeds much easier, as if they came naturally. I mean, what else do heroes do but heroic deeds? All the sacrifices a caregiver must make from day to day became easier.

Shaving my head freed me from the petty pretensions to which I'd become addicted. Suddenly it didn't matter if anyone found me attractive with hair or without hair. I had a cause. I had a purpose beyond self-inflation and exaltation. I felt good contributing to the well-being and healing of a person I loved. I felt useful.

Lastly, being bald was something Marthy and I could experience together. Chemotherapy patients suffer tremendously from the isolation that their condition imposes upon them. No cancer patient would wish cancer upon anyone else, yet it helps to talk to another who is experiencing similar fears, challenges, disappointments, and successes. Marthy and I formed our own support group of two. We discovered a new intimacy by shaving each other's heads.

Caregivers, of course, are not required to shave their heads with their patients any more than patients are required to demand their caregivers share their baldness. If shaving your head is appropriate, you'll know. If you feel obligated to shave your head but don't want to, then don't do it. But if the only reason you don't want to shave your head and share the experience with your patient is due to your vanity, then maybe you should reconsider and do it. You'll never regret it. Hair grows back. Time only moves on. And seeing yourselves bald by choice presents an opportunity to laugh together.

Marthy's first grandchild, Madison, was born less than three months before she entered chemotherapy. For the first year of her life, Madison knew her grandmother as bald. When Marthy completed her therapy, we celebrated with a trip to Hawaii for sixteen days. After we returned, Marthy was anxious to visit her granddaughter again. The moment little Madison saw her grandmother, she pointed at Marthy's new growth of hair and laughed. Where we thought bald was funny, she thought having hair was the comedy.

Beauty is truly in the eye of the beholder, just like humor. Share a shave with your patient and you'll learn that bald can be beautiful in many ways. Discover the liberation of a life without hair and the intimacy of going truly topless with your partner.

Bald is better together. No joke.

Exercises for Chapter Eight

Tell your patient you're thinking of getting a haircut.

Think of how easy it would be not to have to wash your hair.

Count your hats.

Chapter Nine

Caregivers for Caregivers

As much as we all want to save our loved ones, we can't do it alone. We need health professionals to treat our patients and effect a cure. Caregivers are the support team for these professionals, but the support team needs support too. So who supports a support team? Another support team, of course.

Join a caregivers' support group. Don't try to decide whether you need a support group or not. Just do it. The only way to know if you need a support group is to join one and see. If you don't need it, you don't have to stay. If you do need it, you'll know right away.

Remember that while you're making every effort to keep your patient from feeling abandoned and alone, you must make the same effort to keep yourself from feeling abandoned as well. Any oncologist's office can provide you with details about local support groups. If all you can find are groups supporting patients, start your own caregivers' group. Ask a caregiver you know to meet you for coffee. Take a walk together. Talk about the things that bother you, the things you can't share with your patient. You'll be surprised to find how universal your feelings are.

When friends offer to take over for an hour, a day, or a few days, don't refuse them. You need the time off, so take time for yourself. Don't fall into the trap of believing no one can care for your patient as well as you can. Even if it's true, you still need to take care of yourself in order to be able to continue caring for your loved one.

Of course it's true: no one can care for your patient exactly like you do. Each of us is different; each has different tastes, different abilities, and different talents. Don't become upset if your relief caregiver does everything differently than you. Expect it and learn to appreciate it. Consider the differences and try to learn from them. Is a new approach better, worse, or just different? Try to be objective. You might discover a better way to approach your job or simply a new way to peel a carrot. You might also learn that there is no better way to care for your loved one than just the way you have been, which is a valuable lesson in itself.

Don't be afraid to watch and listen. Don't be afraid to let go for a while. Caregivers have needs, too. Don't feel selfish about seeing that your needs are met. Just be sure your relief caregiver is prepared.

After I had been caring for my stepfather Ed for several months without a break, his son Greg arrived from Virginia to take over. I was immensely grateful and eagerly met him at the airport in Portland. On the drive back to the house I realized he hadn't a clue of what he'd stepped into.

"So," Greg said, "how's Dad?"

"You're serious," I answered. "You really don't know?"

"He said he's got emphysema and something like sleep apnea," my stepbrother said.

"He's got five kinds of cancer," I said, gauging my brother's response. "He really didn't tell you?"

Greg shook his head, stunned.

"Lung, kidney, prostate, and bone, in just this past month. Damn, I've forgotten one of them."

Greg stared at me.

"Do you know what a hospice program is?" I asked.

He shook his head again. "Someplace where young people stay when they travel?" he asked.

"That's a hostel," I said. "Hospice is a program of medical care you enter only in the last six months of your life."

"Dad's only got six months to live?" he asked quietly.

"No, your dad entered a hospice program three months ago. We don't know how long he has to live, but it's substantially less than six months now."

"Why didn't he tell me?" Greg struck the dashboard of the car with his fist. "I knew he wasn't doing so good or he wouldn't have asked me to come home."

"Is that all he told you?"

"Yeah. I asked for more details, but he avoided the subject."

"He's got forty-nine medications daily. You've got to be sure he takes them. He needs help getting dressed and into and out of bed. Oh, and the portable toilet. I'll show you when we get to the house."

"The toilet? Can we stop for a drink? I need to think."

"Sure," I said. "I'll only be gone a week. Don't worry. You'll be all right."

I was lying. I could see he wasn't prepared. But I needed a break. I needed to go home and be with my wife, see my sons, see a few friends, pet my cat, sit in the sun, and read and think and not listen for a call from the bedroom down the hall.

I left on a Monday evening. The next day my phone rang. It was my stepbrother.

"We need you back," Greg said. "Mom fell and broke her hip. She's in the hospital and I've got to stay with Dad."

With less than twenty-four hours off after months of caregiving, I was back at it again. Worse, I was convinced that I'd somehow caused the accident by leaving my mother and stepfather in my stepbrother's hands, well intentioned as he might have been.

Three days after I returned, Ed died at home with Greg, my brother Craig, and me. My mother was in the hospital recovering from her surgery. Her Alzheimer's shielded her a little from the loss but not completely. That first night, I slept in a cot next to her bed at the hospital.

After his father's death, Greg went limp emotionally and physically. Day after day he sat in his father's favorite chair and stared out the window. I became enmeshed in my mother's care, moving her from the hospital to a rehabilitation center, visiting and encouraging her, and then transitioning her back to her home without her husband waiting for her. I was convinced I couldn't leave again or something even more awful would befall my patient.

Less than a month later, I found myself a patient in the same emergency room at the same hospital where I'd taken my stepfather so many times and my mother just a few weeks before. The official medical report stated acute pancreatitis and congestive heart failure, but I know the cause was simply stress. I couldn't let go of the duties to my loved ones and became obsessed with those obligations until they nearly drove me into my own grave.

Remember, as a caregiver you have become responsible only for the care and support of your loved one. You are not responsible for your patient's healing or survival. This is the fine line a caregiver must walk, a line I stepped over several times. Without realizing what I was doing, I accepted the responsibility for my loved ones' recoveries. When they died, I failed. Then I accepted the guilt that felt appropriate. Simple grief is hard enough to live with. Guilt-ridden grief is an impossible burden.

Treatment is the doctor's responsibility. Healing is ultimately the job of the patient. Being good to and for the patient is the best you can do.

Don't try to do it alone. Let someone step in and take over for a while. Find someone you can talk to, and then go ahead and complain to him or her. Join a support group. Take time for yourself, and vent your frustrations. If you feel like a martyr, say so. Then find a way not to feel like one. If you feel selfish, admit it. Then do what you need to do for yourself first so that you can do what you must for your loved one later.

There's a reason airlines instruct adults, in case of emergency, to put their own oxygen masks on before they put the masks on their children. Remember to breathe.

EXERCISES FOR CHAPTER NINE

Call someone you trust and complain.

Ask a friend or family member to give you a day off.

Practice taking long, slow breaths—focus on filling your chest.

Do something special every day just for you.

Chapter Ten

Mr. Barleycorn Is Not Your Buddy

When I was caring for my stepfather, Ed, he purchased a small bell like those that once were commonly found on hotel registry desks. He placed it on his nightstand, next to his bed. Rather than calling for assistance, he'd ring that bell.

The sound of Ed's bell carried throughout the house and beyond, into the garage and the gardens. He told me the bell was only for urgent requests, but he rang it often, even if he knew I was farthest from his room and occupied with another task. I could be taking out the garbage and he'd ring just to ask for batteries that lay within his reach. I soon realized that he needed to exert control over a world in which he had none.

I grew to hate that bell.

I began to awaken at night, imagining I'd heard him ring for me. When I'd return to sleep, I'd dream that I heard the bell again. I'd re-awaken and lie quietly, waiting for its tone. When I didn't hear it, I couldn't go back to sleep until I'd crept to his door to make sure he wasn't desperate for assistance. I slept less and less. The less rest I got, the more frequently I dreamed of ringing bells.

The dreams soon grew longer and more detailed. One dream repeated itself night after night. In it, Ed summoned me from my sleep. He had to urinate and struggled to sit up. I prepared the urinal bottle and held it for him as he peed. In my dream, he continued to pee until he filled the bottle and it began to overflow. I had no other bottle with which to replace it. I begged him to stop, but he just smiled sleepily and continued to pee. The urine overflowed out of the bottle, over my hands, my arms, and onto the bed and the carpet. I always awakened wet with a clammy sweat, listening for the bell.

I began to dread going to bed. I'd stay up long after Mom and Ed had retired, watching old movies on television or reading. I began treating myself to a martini after dinner. I discovered that a drink relaxed me after a long day. I doubled the shots and found it relaxed me even more. Within a few weeks, I was treating myself to two double martinis every evening. They helped me sleep, I told my mother and Ed. They hid me from the nightmares, I told myself. It was true: the more I drank, the less I dreamed. Or maybe I remembered less of my dreams.

Ed often couched his requests in terms of my mother's concerns, believing I'd honor her needs over his own.

"Your mother wants chicken for dinner tonight," he might say, though we both knew that with her Alzheimer's, Mom didn't remember if we'd had dinner already or not.

"Your mother is worried about you drinking in the evenings," he said to me one night.

"I understand," I said.

From then on, I kept my bottles in my bedroom. I changed my habits, began to retire earlier. I mixed my drinks at my desk and read or scribbled bad poetry. I changed my drink of choice from gin to vodka, although I disliked the taste. I remembered reading that vodka couldn't be smelled on your breath.

I told myself I hid my drinking to protect my mother and Ed from worrying unnecessarily about me. I told myself they needed to reserve their concerns for themselves. I told myself I was only self-medicating, that I deserved the respite the alcohol gave me after a hard day of cooking, cleaning, changing diapers, taking orders, and not arguing with Ed.

If a day seemed unusually difficult, I began sneaking a drink before dinner. Soon, every day seemed too trying for me. I told myself my drinking was temporary, that I'd quit as soon as the situation improved. I told myself I could handle the alcohol, that it didn't affect me the same as it did others. The truth was that the more I drank, the less it affected me. The less it affected me, the more I drank.

I missed Marthy. I missed my life and my home. I hadn't expected to remain so long as the sole caregiver for my parents. My mother's Alzheimer's continued to progress, and she continued to deteriorate. Watching her lose little pieces of herself day by day wrenched my heart.

Ed's body failed a little more every few days, too. His doctors discovered that his new pains were the result of new cancers. As his strength declined, our arguments diminished commensurately. I discovered that the less difficult he became, the more difficult I found it to care for him. I realized that I did love him after all, after thirty-two years of butting heads, after disagreeing over this and that and everything, after all the hurt and humiliation and anger. I didn't like my mother's husband, but watching him die was still too hard to do sober. So I drank even more.

He died in my arms. I stroked his head and told him that he could go, that I'd take care of Mom for him. I tried to close his eyelids the way you see them do in the movies, but it doesn't work that way. I pressed his lids closed for several minutes with my fingertips, but his left eye just wouldn't stay shut. It stared at me sadly no matter where I stood. Long after his body had been removed from the house, he still fixed me with that lifeless stare.

So I drank. I drank to escape the pain, and to escape the confusion of disliking and loving all at the same time. And I drank to escape the loss of a man with whom I never made peace, but whom I did my best to comfort as he died.

Drinking didn't help. My pain and confusion remained just as intense and were perhaps exacerbated by the alcohol. The more I hurt, the more I drank, and the more I drank, the more I hurt.

Mom had fallen and broken her hip three days before Ed died. I'd seen her to the hospital, then to a convalescent facility, splitting my time between them. With Ed gone, I needed to see her home again and arrange for professional care for her. I began interviewing caregivers. None of them seemed good enough for my mother.

Three weeks later, Marthy drove down from Vashon Island. I'd developed a pain in my chest that wouldn't go away—a sort of cramp, not at all like a heart attack, but bothersome. Marthy said that she didn't like the way I sounded on the phone. Her daughter had just given birth to her first child and had been hospitalized in Seattle with toxemia. Though Marthy was torn, she sensed something was very wrong with me and left the same day for Oregon. To further complicate the situation, her station wagon had developed suspension problems, so she drove to a hotel in Tacoma and rented a car.

I was surprised and embarrassed by her concern for me.

"I'll just go to bed," I told her when she arrived. "If the pain's not better by morning, I'll see a doctor."

She then told me the magic words every woman must say to a man sometime: "If you don't let me take you," she insisted, "I'll dial 9-1-1 and totally embarrass you."

By the time we reached the hospital, I couldn't catch my breath. The pain had become a spear of molten metal driven through my body.

When I reached the emergency room, two nurses started morphine intravenously in both my arms simultaneously. I watched in amazement.

"Is this serious?" I asked the attending physician.

She was a young woman with dark, combative eyes.

"Are you kidding, bub?" she answered. "In another hour, you wouldn't be here."

The diagnosis was congestive heart failure, acute pancreatitis, acute inflammation of the gall bladder, and acute gastritis. An MRI revealed that a growth the size of a softball had consumed most of my pancreas, had grown through my stomach, and was pressing on my heart. They drained several quarts of fluid from my chest cavity. I was on a Demerol drip for two weeks, during which I suffered the wildest hallucinations imaginable. A month later, the growth and most of what was left of my pancreas were surgically removed. I was too weak to take two steps without resting, but I was alive.

My doctor told me I could have no more alcohol, no fatty foods, no acidic fruits or vegetables, no peppers, no caffeine, and no simple sugars. I haven't had a drink since the day Marthy drove me to the hospital, but I have to sneak a spoonful of peanut butter every now and then. And, I hope that chocolate is food for the soul, because it might kill me in the end. I'm only human.

If you are a caregiver for a chemotherapy patient, you are facing some of the most difficult times of your life. Heed my experience. No matter how hard your life becomes, no matter how much you hurt and feel you need to hide, please don't drink. Alcohol will not help you deal with your fear or pain. Alcohol only makes everything worse. Booze is a buddy who will turn on you and steal all you have—your money, your loved ones, your self-respect, and your very soul.

If the pain of witnessing your patient's fight becomes too great for you, ask for help. If you're already using alcohol as a support mechanism, call someone you can trust. Be honest with yourself and your loved ones about how much you drink. If you have no one to turn to, look in the phone book. Alcoholics Anonymous lists phone numbers you can call anywhere in the world. Don't worry about what anyone thinks of you. Judgment isn't what's offered, only help.

Being a caregiver for a chemo patient often feels lonely, but you should remember that you are never alone. You are surrounded by people who are willing to help, including many you may not have even met yet. People will stay with you much longer than John Barleycorn. Turn to the people who love you instead of the bottle. Take a hug instead of a hit. Give those who love you a chance, and you will save yourself as well as your patient.

Please.

EXERCISES FOR CHAPTER TEN

Call a friend instead of pouring a drink.

Remind yourself that the one whose respect you need most is the one you see everyday in the mirror.

Be naughty and sneak a rootbeer float to bed tonight.

Chapter Eleven

And What's Up with Huckleberry Bushes and Cedar Stumps?

You don't tell bus driver jokes to a proctologists' convention. Similarly, you might fall flat with their jokes regarding posterior elevations if you tried to entertain a group of Martha Stewart devotees. Where the line "And what's up with huckleberry bushes and cedar stumps?" might give rise to chuckles when delivered to a dinner honoring foresters, a room filled with chefs might be left wondering what berries have to do with dispelling moths from closets. Just as with any amusement, cancer humor is specific to the audience.

As a caregiver, don't expect every joke you find funny to fall on appreciative ears. Conversely, don't expect to see humor in whatever causes your patient to laugh out loud. And never be surprised if those outside your patient-caregiver relationship have no idea at all what you are both laughing about.

Marthy saw an extraterrestrial on a television series called *The Outer Limits*. The alien was small, slender, and very nearly translucent. Its slight body was absolutely hairless, with a large head and luminous dark eyes. She pointed it out to me, saying it was exactly what she thought she looked like.

Months later, we found ourselves in Issaquah, Washington, after losing our way on a delightful day of driving through the Cascade foothills looking for a small café that we discovered had gone out of business years before. We stopped to shop in a toy store for a gift for Marthy's granddaughter. As we browsed among plastic dinosaurs and kites, I discovered a reproduction of the extraterrestrial we'd seen on television. It stood with arms outstretched as if in greeting—three elongated fingers on each hand, large eyes dark and luminous. It was not only nearly translucent but phosphorescent as well and glowed in the dark. I bought it for her, and she cradled it in her lap, laughing all the way home.

The doll did resemble Marthy. Without hair or any cell regeneration, her skin had become nearly as translucent as the doll's. I used to study her in the dusk of our evening bedroom, convinced that she did indeed glow as well. But, however much Marthy resembled the doll, I couldn't share the amusement she derived from it.

One day she took the doll to a Taxol treatment at the Tumor Institute in Seattle. She explained to Dr. Goodman that she thought the chemo made her look like an extraterrestrial and pulled the doll out of her bag as proof. He gave her a sheepish grin but seemed genuinely confused by her delight.

As we left Dr. Goodman's office, we bumped into a friend who had been diagnosed with breast cancer several months after Marthy. We sat and chatted with her while she waited for her appointment. During the course of the conversation, another chemo patient joined us. Marthy pulled the doll out of her bag and began the explanation of how she thought she resembled the creature, but they never let her finish. All I could do was sit and watch as all three of them laughed until they cried.

Now the doll stands on the dresser in our bedroom, where I can see its ghostly glow after we turn the lights out. Marthy still gets a kick out of looking at it, and though I remember the resemblance, I still don't understand the humor. It's enough for me to see Marthy laugh. It's her way of reminding herself to spit in the eye of the Universe.

Some humor you can share with your patient and some you can't. You won't know which it will be until it happens. Sharing a laugh about an inside joke with your patient creates a bond others will never comprehend.

Our friend Beth suffered for seven years, stamping out one kind of cancer just to see it erupt in another part of her body as a different kind. Finally the doctors told her to go home, because there was nothing more they could do. Her first grandchild had been born just months before, and both Beth and her husband Chuck found great joy playing with her.

Shortly after the doctors sent her home, Beth was sitting in front of the fire one evening with her husband. She seemed preoccupied and distant—staring absently into the fire. Chuck asked her what was bothering her, fearful of her answer, but obligated to ask anyway.

"I made a mistake," she said quietly. "A big mistake."

"What is it?" he asked anxiously. "Tell me and I'll fix it."

"You can't fix this one," she said.

"Tell me anyway," he urged her, thinking she'd said something rude or sent the wrong card to one of their daughters.

"Remember when I was first diagnosed with cancer?" she answered. "Remember they asked me what I wanted?"

"Yes," he said.

"I said I wanted to live long enough to see my first grandchild born."

"I remember," he said. "And you did that; our grandchild is beautiful. What's the mistake?"

"I should have said 'grandchildren'."

They looked at each other for a moment and then burst into laughter. They laughed on and off about that conversation for the next several weeks. Most who hear their story see no humor in it, only tender tragedy. To those who have never faced death, the humor must appear macabre. To Beth and Chuck, it provided the relief they needed in the darkest of their hours.

No matter how dark the future appears, don't ever be afraid to laugh. Laughter defeats fear. It's also good for digestion, unless it makes the milk and cookies come out your nose.

EXERCISES FOR CHAPTER ELEVEN

Make up a funny name for something your patient is sensitive about.

Buy a book of funny one-liners.

Never forget: People without feet don't need shoes.

Chapter Twelve

Cleaning the Range

A few years ago, my son returned from a couple of years in Europe. With him he brought two suitcases, a large box, too many memories, too few photos, and a six-foot-two Swedish bombshell. He'd met Malin on the island of Santorini in Greece, and they'd traveled most of Europe together, landing in London for six months before coming home to the United States. She was twenty-one, beautiful, and full of youthful opinions, most of them inviolably Swedish. The first morning they were in my house, I prepared a scramble of eggs, spinach, garlic, and Kasseri cheese while they slept late. I was grating the Kasseri when Malin stumbled sleepily into the kitchen.

"You're slicing the cheese wrong," she said without a good morning preface.

I was a little taken back. I hadn't known this young woman for more than twelve hours.

"Do you even know what I'm making?" I asked.

"Doesn't matter," she shrugged and ate a couple of squiggles of Kasseri. "In Sweden, we slice the cheese—how do you say it—length-long."

"Is how you do something in Sweden always the only way?" I teased her.

"Obviously the best way," she said and smiled. "Here, let me show you."

"I know how to slice cheese 'length-long'," I said. "I want the cheese grated so it will melt evenly in the scramble."

"You Americans," she pouted, "always have to have your own way."

Over the next three months, we had several such conversations. Swedish ways were always the best, and any time I suggested she simply observe how things were done in our household, she'd pout about how we Americans always had to have everything our way. She was obviously quite homesick, but when I suggested that might be the case, she worried that I wanted her to leave. I never brought up the subject again.

She was a sweet girl with an enormous heart and an equally enormous capacity for hard work. I had just purchased a house in Issaquah, Washington, twenty miles into the Cascade Mountains, and was preparing to move for the first time in fourteen years. Anyone who has settled anywhere for any length of time understands how many possessions one can accumulate. My closets were crammed with keepsakes, my basement was stuffed, and my car barely squeezed into my garage due to the boxes of valuables stacked along the walls. I wouldn't call myself a packrat. I simply develop attachments easily—to broken tennis rackets, old boots, rocks picked up on ocean beaches, and scraps of buildings I intend to use somewhere someday.

Where my sons were respectful, Malin was ruthless in helping me sort through the accumulation. If it wasn't for her, I might still be in Ballard, hopelessly mired in my belongings.

Just a few days before the moving date, she asked me to leave the final cleaning of the kitchen to her.

"It's not that you're not clean," she told me tactfully. "Just that Americans aren't as clean as we Swedes."

I gratefully turned the entire chore over to her, with one admonishment. The electric range was old and tarnished. I'd replaced the burners and essential parts as they had expired over the years, but the burner rings and other parts that had once been bright and polished when the appliance was new were no longer shining. Our landlord had told me not to bother cleaning the range, that he was going to buy a new one as a gift to his daughter and her husband, the next tenants in line for the house.

"Don't clean the range," I told Malin. "Bob's going to buy a new one for his daughter."

The next day my sons and I had errands that took us out and about for the entire afternoon. When we left, Malin was ardently attacking the sink and kitchen counters with cleansers. When we returned just before suppertime, she was finishing the range.

"I thought you weren't going to clean the range," I said diplomatically.

"I know," she said, stepping back to admire her work. "But doesn't it look great?"

It did indeed look great. It looked brand new.

"But Bob's just going to throw it away, anyway," I protested.

"At least it will look great when he throws it away," she said with pride. "And besides, the hours were going to pass whether I cleaned it or not. I could have spent the time watching television, but now I've accomplished something."

I looked at the pride in her eyes and at the shining electric range. I recognized the wisdom in her words.

Years before, when my brother Chris relapsed, the statistics regarding possible recovery were bleak. Few had ever come back from a recurrence of a lymphoma like his. Without a matched donor and without having harvested his own marrow while he was in remission, the prospect of a bone marrow transplant seemed painfully futile. He didn't want to fight any longer. He was so fatigued by four years of chemo and radiation that he simply wanted to lie down and rest.

I remember discussing the options with him. Any chance he had was slim or none. Still, I was reluctant to let him go, so I cajoled him and appealed to his sense of family.

"We made a pact," I reminded him. "We promised each other to never leave any stone unturned."

"I know," he said, "but it's no use. I can't beat it."

"Then you have to fight for the family," I said. "If you don't, we'll always wonder 'what if?' We'll always wonder if there was something else we could have done to save you."

I'll never know if it was my arguments, his wife's, our sister's, our other brother's, our mother's, or his own, but he changed his mind and chose to try a bone marrow transplant.

It didn't work. The lymphoma claimed him anyway, but the transplant did grant him another year of life during which he found a lot to laugh about, a lot to love, and witnessed at least the beginnings of his only child, Erica, who was born two months after he died.

That year was going to pass anyway. I'm sure he was glad it passed with him along for the ride, no matter how bumpy the road at times.

And the electric range? Bob never threw it away. Malin did such a wonderful job restoring it, he gave it to his daughter and her husband. I believe they're baking muffins in that old stove to this day.

EXERCISES FOR CHAPTER TWELVE

Whenever you feel despair, clean your stove.

Bake something really sloppy to soil your stove again.

Begin a long-term project with your patient.

Take a Swedish cooking class.

Try cutting cheese "length-long."

Chapter Thirteen

Patience Is Your Job, Not Your Patient's

During the months I cared for my stepfather, Ed, I learned several important lessons I never expected to discover. I'd never taken care of a patient who denied he was going to die. That alone posed several challenges, but I'm still assimilating and figuring out the biggest lesson of all. I'm not sure how to write about it or even if I should, because I believe I'll still be sorting it out for the rest of my days.

As hard as it is to take care of someone you love as he or she fights for life, it's still easier than taking care of someone you don't love. When you're caring for someone you don't love, you want to walk away and let someone else, anyone else, do it for you. But you don't, because there isn't anyone else: if there was, you wouldn't be there. And you don't because you know that everyone deserves care, even the most difficult of patients—maybe, especially the most difficult patients. A patient who is being difficult may be having a harder time dealing with the situation than one who is easy to love, easy to care for, and easy to be around. The crankier a patient, the more he or she may need you.

I took care of Ed during his final months not because of my affection for him, but because I love my mother. Mom loved Ed very much, but because she had Alzheimer's disease, could not care for him herself. Ed and I had never really gotten along, but over the thirty-two years he was married to my mother, we had achieved a sort of uneasy truce. He was apologetic when Mom had called me to stay with them after he'd been taken to the hospital unexpectedly. Unexpectedly for any of the rest of us in the family because he'd neglected to tell any of us that he had cancers. He'd smoked for more than fifty years and was reluctant to admit that all our admonishments regarding the health risks had been correct. He was reluctant to ever admit he was wrong about anything, so he told us he had a "little emphysema." His little emphysema turned out to be five kinds of cancer, starting with his lungs.

"I'll only need you a week," he told me when I picked him up at the hospital.

Three months later he died at home in my arms. In between those two events we came to accept, if not actually like, one another. I found it difficult to care for someone who was so insecure and controlling that he wouldn't tell me which way to turn on the drive to his doctor's office until we were hard upon the intersection.

"Put your signal on now," he commanded me.

"Which way?" I asked.

"Right! Right! You're not even in the right lane. Damn it, now you've missed the turn," he shouted.

"Why not just tell me where we're going and let me get us there?" I asked him.

He never had an answer, but I suspect he simply needed to feel in control of something, anything, once he could no longer control his destiny on a grander scale.

Confronting a patient about such insecurities does not help. I became angry when Ed didn't trust me to make his soft-boiled egg the way he asked. He wanted me to boil the water a full minute before I put the egg in the pan, then set the timer for three minutes, then remove the pan from the heat and time another minute on my watch before placing the egg in a bowl. It wasn't the exacting nature of his request that bothered me; it was that he felt it necessary to stand next to me, timing me on his watch as I timed his eggs, to ensure that I followed his directions to the letter.

"You can't even trust me to make a soft-boiled egg the way you ask," I complained to him.

"How else will I know you did it right?" he replied.

"If you can't tell by how it tastes, what do you care?" I answered.

"You could fool me and I'd never know," he said.

One day I got up earlier than usual and hard-boiled an egg. That morning he watched me time his egg and then, satisfied, sat down to enjoy his breakfast. I switched eggs on the way to the table and set his bowl before him. When he cracked the shell of the hard-boiled egg, he started chuckling. He never watched me prepare his eggs again.

Ed seemed to become most difficult whenever he needed me most. For instance, when he used his portable toilet during the night, he'd be crankier than usual in the morning when he rang his bell to summon me. He'd avoid my eyes and complain about something other than the job I was performing. One morning, instead of sneaking the bucket out quickly, I swung it around the bedroom like a dancing partner.

"Only poop," I sang to the tune of "Only You," "can make the world go 'round . . . Only poop, can make that awful sound . . . Only poop and poop alone, can wrinkle my nose like this, and fill the bucket with its companion, piss . . . "

Despite my lurid lyrics and inability to carry a tune, Ed and Mom doubled with laughter. Ed was never cranky again when he called me into his bedroom to empty the bucket. Maybe he was simply afraid I might burst into another song of dubious color, but I like to think it was because he was no longer embarrassed by it.

Try to remember that when your patient is being most difficult, it usually isn't about you at all. Try to realize that when your patient is most fearful, embarrassed, or uncomfortable is when he or she will be the most difficult. And patients are difficult when they need you the most.

Don't meet frustration and anger with frustration and anger. You can't treat fear with fear. If your patient is short-tempered or abrupt, try not to respond in kind.

Remember to breathe before you respond. And remember that humor is the great liberator. Use humor when you feel like being angry or abrupt. You'll discover yourself liberated along with your patient. And never forget that being patient is your job, not your patient's.

EXERCISES FOR CHAPTER THIRTEEN

Make up a silly song to sing for your patient.

Get a bucket to put on your head when you feel angry.

If your patient becomes angry, pass the bucket.

Chapter Fourteen

Re-state to Clarify, Align to Deflect

Never take an attack personally. Most attacks have nothing to do with the caregiver or the quality of care given. Most attacks have everything to do with fear. The patient may need to lash out in self-defense, but without a physical body to hit, cancer can be an elusive opponent.

Caregivers, however, are not elusive. Caregivers are quite handy and should expect to become emotional punching bags at times. This is one area where humor doesn't help until later, sometimes much later. Logic is no aid either, and caregivers might be well advised not to offer any. When dealing with fear, presenting logical solutions can be like pouring gasoline on a fire. We usually don't want solutions when we're upset; we just want someone to listen.

As I mentioned in an earlier chapter, chemotherapy is a roller coaster, and sometimes it helps to scream on the way down. Sometimes, it helps to have someone to scream at as well, and if you're the caregiver, you're it. If you can see it coming, put on your best emotional asbestos suit. Take the first couple of blasts and then back away. Give your patient time to regain control. Go for a walk or a drive. Don't tell the patient anything inflammatory before you leave. Never say you're leaving because he or she has become irrational. That response is certain to incite further irrationality.

Tell your patient you need time to think about what he or she has said. Or say you need to be alone to understand what you've done to elicit the attack. Never accept the blame unless you truly believe it's your fault. Never assign the blame to someone else under any conditions, even if you're certain you know where the fault lies. And never stand toe to toe with your patient in a shouting match. It's always a competition without any winners.

Being burned by a loved one is never fun, but neither is having cancer. Never take a burning personally. Retreat, heal your blisters, remind yourself why you're there in the first place, and return after the ashes have cooled.

If you find yourself in a situation where you cannot back away, remember these two rules: Restate to clarify. Align to deflect.

When someone attacks you verbally, the charge is rarely rational. An irrational attack is particularly hurtful and can make a caregiver feel unappreciated—the worst of all sins a patient can commit. If you cannot retreat from an irrational attack, restate it in similar words so the patient can hear for himself or herself what has been said. In extreme cases, you might have to restate the attack in exactly the same words to avoid denial and repetitive attacks by the patient.

Often, simply restating the attack blunts the patient's anger. The reason any of us strike out at loved ones is rarely for the reasons we think at the time. Once we hear what we've said, we're usually appalled at ourselves, and become apologetic.

"You don't love me!" someone might have said to me. "You didn't come to bed when I did."

"Let me see if I understand you clearly," I might have replied. "You think I don't love you because I'm staying up later to answer our e-mail?"

I didn't really respond in this manner, but I should have. Instead, I puffed out my chest and, in my best imitation of an unfairly importuned little boy, responded with something as eloquent as, "Oh yeah? Well, this really makes me want to come to bed!"

Had I responded by restating the attack, the argument probably would have ended right there. Instead it ended when she decided she couldn't live with someone who didn't care enough about her to come to bed at the same time. She slammed the door on her way to stay with her daughter.

Should your patient continue the attack after you've restated the charges, the next step is to align yourself with him or her. Ask your patient if he or she is certain that what was said is really how your patient feels. If the answer is yes, then tell your patient that you understand. Say that you think you might feel the same way if you were in the same position. Remind your patient that you are both on the same side. We can't stay mad at someone who is agreeing with us.

"I understand how you might feel that way," I could have responded to the attack over different bedtimes. "Maybe I should have asked if you wanted to talk before you went to sleep. Give me a minute to brush my teeth. I'll be right there."

If the attack continues, ask your patient how a solution might be found. If your patient cannot come up with a solution, offer some options casually as questions, always keeping him or her engaged. Never dictate. Never offer only one solution, and never recommend a particular solution. Offer several choices and allow the patient to select one or more he or she thinks is appropriate. Discuss the solutions and different ways to implement them. Keep the patient involved.

"You don't feel like talking now?" I could have said. "Maybe we should just spend some quiet time together?"

If the response continues to be negative, continue the involvement.

"Would you like me to read to you instead? How about some cocoa? I know you like hot chocolate. Are you cold?"

The key is to make sure your patient feels in control. Not so strangely, when we feel out of control is when we're most likely to act out of control. A chemotherapy patient has precious little control of his or her destiny.

Once a dialogue is established, remember to listen. Try not to interrupt. Let your patient say what he or she needs to say. Sometimes someone who feels at the whim of dark and evil forces like cancers will act a little cranky. Go figure.

EXERCISES FOR CHAPTER FOURTEEN

Look into a mirror and pretend you are the one with cancer.

Challenge your patient to a card game and be sure to lose.

Give your patient a menu from which he or she can select meals.

Allow your patient to select your wardrobe one day each week.

Chapter Fifteen

Sometimes Being There Is More Important Than Being Right

There comes a time in everyone's life when a little lie is better than the truth. We've all told little white lies. For instance, when Marthy was at her nadir, the lowest point in her chemotherapy (both physically and emotionally), she feared that I didn't find her attractive any longer.

"How can you look at me," she worried. "I'm a hairless worm, no eyelashes, no eyebrows, not a hair on my whole body. Not even in my nose."

"You're more beautiful than you've ever been," I lied. "In some cultures the women shave their bodies to make them more attractive."

"You're lying," she laughed. "But I like it. Keep it up."

"In fact, I understand there are places right here in this country where I'd have to pay big bucks to look at an exotic dancer who went to a lot of trouble to become as attractive," I continued.

"Okay, that's enough," she said. "You're digging deep now."

As a caregiver, there will be times when you'll find yourself lying. Those will be the times when a lie is not only easier than the truth but also better, for both parties, than a factual response.

Over the seven years Beth battled her cancers, there were several times she found herself dwindling away without hope of recovery. Each time, as she lay in her bed, certain she was near expiration, she'd turn to her husband Chuck—her caregiver, her soul mate, and her trusted partner.

"Am I dying?" she'd ask him.

Even though he sincerely believed she was dying every time she would ask, he'd take her hand, look her straight in the eye, and lie.

"No," he'd say. "You just have to manage your pain better and get more fluids in you."

She'd study his face and then sigh.

"Okay," she'd say.

She'd do it, too. She'd do whatever he said would save her. And then she'd rebound. He tells me that he never knew the solutions to her medical situations. He wasn't offering solutions, you see; he was offering hope. Beth trusted him and though she never told him whether or not she believed his remedies, she followed his advice. She followed his hope. Simply believing she could rebound made all the difference.

Of course, telling the truth is the best course most of the time. We all try to be honest, but be prepared for those times when telling a little lie won't hurt. And sometimes telling a big lie will be better than telling a little truth.

Trust your instincts. You'll know when it's the right time to be honest and when it isn't. Don't be afraid to lie when the time is right. Your presence with your patient is more important than always telling the truth.

Be present. Offer hope to your patient. Lie when you need to and do it with a straight face and a pure heart. Maybe saying things you hope are true isn't really lying after all.

EXERCISES FOR CHAPTER FIFTEEN

Go sit next to your patient for no reason at all.

Plan a vacation to celebrate the end of chemotherapy.

Practice telling three little lies a day.

Chapter Sixteen

Looking for Four-Leaf Clovers or Pebbling the Walk

There was a time when I felt guilty if I wasted any hours of my day. I remember telling my kids I wished I didn't have to sleep at all, that I considered sleeping to be a waste of time.

"Think how much more we could do if we didn't have to sleep," I remember saying.

When my little brother Chris was first diagnosed with lymphoma, I had an office in Pioneer Square in Seattle. My public relations and advertising business was my life. I went out to dinner more times a week than I didn't; chatted up more people, told more jokes, and spent more time running in circles than I spent sitting and thinking.

"Come talk with me," Chris would say.

"Can't," I'd say, "got an appointment for a brochure." Or, "Have to meet some people at Ray's." Or, "Gonna be all night in the darkroom printing a big order." There was always something more important.

I never seemed to find the time to sit and contemplate our lives. I was too busy living mine, I thought, to sit and think about it. Too busy doing it to talk about it.

"It's business," I'd explain as if that justified anything.

As time grew short for my brother, he entreated me to spend more with him. As I watched him fail and waste away, I increasingly put my business aside. One day, the doctors said there wasn't anything more they could do.

"Go home and die," they told him. They weren't being cold or heartless, but compassionate, hoping their honesty would give him time to arrange his affairs and be with his loved ones.

After that, I found a lot more time to be with Chris. Other members of our family and some of his friends, however, did not. In an apparent contradiction, once they knew he had only a short time to live, people who had previously made time for him suddenly became too busy to visit. Chris and I talked about this phenomenon.

"There's no room for denial any longer. They can't face what's happening," Chris said. "You can't blame them."

He couldn't blame them but I could. They were missing their last chances to be with him, and no one knew better than I the guilt they would soon be feeling. Once he was gone, each and every one of them mentioned to me their regrets for not seeing more of him when they could.

The time to run away and hide is never when time is short. Nor is it the time to fill your days with frantic activity. Oddly enough, when time is short is the best time to waste time, to idle afternoons away doing absolutely nothing productive at all—nothing but spending time together.

Chris and I spent many of his last days sitting in the sun alongside Lake Washington. We had no agenda, just talked about everything and nothing at all. Some days we lay on the lawn and looked for four-leaf clovers. Always the scientist, he told me the odds against a clover developing four leaves and the odds against anyone actually finding one. I didn't argue with him and am quite sure he was correct. He was, after all, a professor from Dartmouth and usually right about all things empirical.

Instead, I simply bent down and picked a four-leaf clover for him.

"You can't do that," he said.

Then he bent and picked one.

We didn't keep all that we found; once we took one, we rarely plucked any of the others we discovered. But we did spend hours looking for them. We would just lie in the grass and talk and look for four-leaf clovers. Of all the things I did with my brother during the thirty-eight years of his life, the days we idled away doing nothing except talking and looking for four-leaf clovers are among the most memorable.

My sister Karen failed more rapidly in her battle with lymphoma than did Chris. I tried to spend as much time as possible with her but found that living in different cities interfered. I spent half of each week at home near Seattle, attending to my business, and the other half in Portland, sitting with her in her house overlooking her garden.

Her cancer took a different twist than our brother's had. Karen's paralyzed her. It confined her to a hospital bed we had brought to her home. We sat and talked and watched summer turn to fall beyond her windows.

While Karen had been in remission several months earlier, our entire family had gathered at Newport, Oregon, to celebrate our mother's seventy-fifth birthday. The month had been May, the weather warm even for spring, and we walked the ocean beaches the way children do, searching for agates and flying kites.

My mother approached me on the beach that trip and announced she'd never found an agate. I told her I'd find her one. Minutes later I picked up the largest agate I'd ever seen. The stone was irregular, not smoothly polished, but the size of a baseball.

Karen approached me then, drawing me off to one side.

"I've never found an agate either," she confided. "But it doesn't have to be as big as Mom's."

"You don't need me to find you an agate," I told her. "All you have to do is believe. Believe, and stop, and look down."

We stopped walking and looked down. At our feet lay an agate, a large agate, though not as large as the one I'd found for Mom. This stone was round and smoothly polished.

"But you can't do that," she said, delighted.

Then she bent and picked up another.

Those final days overlooking her garden, we talked about the agates we'd found on the beach that day.

"Life is like agates," my sister opined. "You only find what you look for, and you only look for what you'll find."

When Marthy faced her surgeries and consequent chemotherapies, my experiences with my brother and sister were not forgotten. We live in a small cottage surrounded by what I like to call an "island-lawn." An island-lawn increases and decreases in size depending upon the season. You cut an island-lawn by mowing in one direction until you hit something, and then mowing in another until you hit something else. One problem with an island lawn is it is very hard to tell where it begins and where it ends. Particularly in the front of the house, where the bare earth of our driveway sort of peters out into the fringes of the lawn, and a bit of a beaten track leads to our front door.

In an effort to provide some sense of presentation to the front of the house, Marthy and I lined the path with large rocks that we'd uncovered around the property during walks and gardening. In a fit of inspiration that was short on foresight, we decided to fill the path with pretty little stones we picked up off the beach on our strolls. Our beach is a fifteen-minute walk down a very steep hill through huckleberries, madrone, salal, and Oregon grape, alder, and salmonberry thickets and nettles. While a fifteen-minute run down the hill with an empty backpack is invigorating, once twenty pounds of pretty beach pebbles have found their way into the pack, the climb back up becomes thirty to forty minutes of acerbic aerobic exercise. The adjective "acerbic" refers, of course, to the language of the backpacker, not the exercise.

So we expanded our territory to include various beaches on the island to which we could drive. The discipline of strolling the beaches of Vashon Island, seeking pretty beach pebbles for our path, became a metaphor for all that was meaningful in our lives. Spending time together, walking the waterline, scheduling our outings by the moon and tides, and returning with a sack of treasures, felt basic to the best of existence—more than survival, far beyond simply gathering food and fuel for our shelter. Piles of wave-smoothed white quartz, the occasional agate, green gneiss, and speckled pink and gray granite became our four-leaf clovers. As we pebbled the walk to our front door, we talked, cried, and laughed together.

I doubt anyone else cares about our pastime; like the search for four-leaf clovers, pebbling our walk accomplished nothing much for anyone but us. Those who'd see us collecting the stones on the various beaches around the island probably wondered if we were, you know, all together. What they may never know, and what is the real pity, is just how much we truly are together.

None of us can know just how much time we have left in this physical reality. We all spend entirely too much time running around as if tomorrow will be our last day. We need to waste more time doing nothing in particular and something momentous all at the same time. Like looking for four-leaf clovers, picking agates off the sand, or pebbling our walks with our loved ones.

So stop, right now, as you're reading this. Take a long, slow breath. Look around. The best that life has to offer is right here, next to you, within your reach. Don't search for something special; this kind of magic only happens when you're not looking too hard for it. Let it come to you. It might be a four-leaf clover, an agate, a bit of white quartz, spending an hour in the sun with a loved one, or doing nothing in particular except living.

EXERCISES FOR CHAPTER SIXTEEN

Find a patch of clover and lie in it.

Take a walk on a beach.

Stop and look down.

Take a small treasure home, especially if it's a memory.

Chapter Seventeen

Resistance without Effort

The concept of resisting by not resisting is very Buddhist, very Christian, and certainly very Jewish. Maybe it's simply very spiritual because it demands a lot of faith. Yet resistance without effort is actually older than religions.

Long before Homo sapiens walked this planet, the physical laws of the Universe demanded that every action be met with an equal and opposite reaction. This means that when we resist, we give whatever it is we are resisting strength equal to our own. With regard to chemotherapy, when we resist we give our opponent even more strength than we ourselves possess since stamina is in short supply.

I first learned of resistance without effort as a child growing up on my parents' farm. We lived on a bluff high above Puget Sound with our own water system, a collection of springs deep in the woods nearly to the beach below our house. My father never seemed to get around to packing the sleeves of the pump until after dark on a cold night.

Because I was the oldest son, Dad always took me with him. Not because I was of any assistance, but for the company; perhaps I was a witness to his efforts. On these evenings, I always began to shiver, sitting on the damp moss of a maple limb above the flume, handing him tools.

Dad was a large man and rarely wore more than a single sweatshirt, no matter what the weather. He'd look at me huddling against the wind and he'd laugh.

"Don't give in to it," he'd say. "It just makes you colder. Throw your shoulders back and your chest out. Embrace the wind; you can't hide from it anyway."

The first time I followed his advice, I was surprised to discover he was right. It worked. By accepting the cold, I didn't feel it as much. But, the knowledge that his approach worked wasn't enough to help me do it every time I felt cold. I'd continue to shiver until he'd remind me and only then would I throw back my shoulders and rediscover the truth in his advice. I can't say why I didn't remember to do it each time without being reminded. Maybe because cold, like fear, creeps up on us, gets hold of us a little at a time, until we're shivering without being aware that we are.

Now that Dad is gone, I have to remember for myself whenever I become cold or afraid. Maybe I needed his reminders simply because I knew he would remind me. Maybe, as caregivers, we become parents of sorts to our patients, even if they are our own parents, and maybe one of our roles as caregivers is to offer the reminders.

Something about being a patient demands that we accept being cared for. When we give in to needing care, somehow we need more, rely on our caregivers for more, and become more dependent upon them. Maybe giving in to becoming dependent upon our caregivers is all part of the retreat that means progress. Perhaps the best way to brace yourself against the fear of cancer is not by resisting it but by accepting it. It's a fine line we have to draw, where resistance has more to do with fear, and acceptance more to do with courage.

Feel the wind of fear; don't hide from it. Talk to your patient openly about what you can do to help him or her avoid shivering. Help your patient accept having cancer without succumbing to it. To acknowledge a presence does not mean one must surrender to it. But to hide from anything is to be conquered. Before we can defeat an opponent, we have to face him. David had to stand before Goliath before he could cast a stone. I suspect he must have found something funny about standing up to such a giant. I also suspect he laughed before he threw his small stone.

EXERCISES FOR CHAPTER SEVENTEEN

Write down what you fear and why you fear it.

Select the fears you can change.

Identify the fears you can't change.

Light a match and burn the list.

Get yourself a chinese finger puzzle.

Go outside without a coat and feel the wind without giving in
   to it.

Chapter Eighteen

Becoming the Eye
of the Hurricane

Taxol chemotherapy involves a high risk of anaphylactic shock. The first infusions are administered slowly, over a twenty- to twenty-four-hour period, to reduce the chance of reaction. Patients are commonly hospitalized overnight to ensure their safety should such a reaction occur.

When Marthy received her first Taxol treatment, I asked if I could stay with her for the duration. Of course, I was told, but cots were in short supply at the hospital that day. Since we happened to be assigned to a two-bed room, the nurses told me to simply slip into the adjoining bed and not to tell anyone. It was against the rules.

Marthy's mother had given her a new nightgown just for the occasion. I'd expected to sleep in a chair so I'd brought no bedclothes. A nurse thoughtfully brought me a pair of patient's pajamas.

Marthy and I hypothesized about the possibility of hospital personnel coming in early while I was still asleep and confusing me for another patient. I had shaved my head with her when she began losing her hair, so I could have passed for a chemotherapy patient, too. I would probably awake to find other body parts shaved in preparation for surgery, we joked.

The steroids they gave Marthy as preparation for the Taxol made her restless. Although we checked into the hospital in the middle of the afternoon, we didn't drop off to sleep until after three in the morning. I awoke an hour later not to candy stripers lathering me with shaving cream but to Marthy talking on the intercom. Because each bed is provided with a privacy curtain, I couldn't see her from my position. I heard her suggest that someone come in to see for himself what her problem was. I pulled back the curtain and nearly fell out of bed.

What greeted me was worse than anything I could have imagined. My sweet Marthy was sitting up in her bed holding her new nightgown across her lap as if she were collecting apples. But it wasn't apples that filled her lap; it was a large pool of blood. Blood covered her face, her hands, and her arms and legs. The bedclothes and pillow were soaked and a great pool was spreading on the floor. I was stunned, speechless.

She smiled at me.

"The connection between the tubing and my IV came apart," she said.

I shook my head, refusing to process the image.

She held up her bloody arms, looked at them, and laughed.

"Good thing my color is red," she said.

I am still amazed at her ability to find humor in waking to find herself covered in blood.

For the next hour we watched a team of nurses clean up the mess. They wore plastic aprons, long gloves, and full masks due to the toxicity of the chemotherapy. Thankfully, the siphoning of blood and leaking of Taxol had been slow, so very little chemical had spilled onto Marthy. A nurse took her into the bathroom to shower and change. When they were done and she was tucked safely back into bed, her new tubing and connections taped securely in place, she announced she was hungry.

"I'm ravenous," she said.

"Order anything you like," her nurse replied. "You can get anything you want from the cafeteria, twenty-four hours a day."

"Jell-O," Marthy said. "I want some cherry Jell-O."

"No, seriously," the nurse said, "anything you like."

"She's serious," I said. Marthy likes Jell-O. She's probably the only patient ever admitted to any hospital who actually looks forward to getting her ration of Jell-O.

They told her the phone number, helped her dial it, and she ordered her snack.

"I'd like four cups of Jell-O," she said. "Cherry Jell-O."

Twenty minutes later a young woman crept in the door with her eyes averted, slipped a tray onto Marthy's table, and nearly made it out of the room before I stopped her.

"Wait a minute," I said. "What's this?"

"Jelly," the girl said timidly. "Four cups of cherry jelly, just like she asked."

The kitchen couldn't believe that anyone would ever order Jell-O in a hospital and had sent jelly instead.

We still laugh at the jelly delivery, though no one else seems to appreciate the joke. Coming so hard on the heels of the bloody episode, the jelly confusion seems oddly perfect, sublimely ridiculous. Our friends see only the blood and the horror of awakening to such a nightmare. For us, the bloodletting is eclipsed by the jelly miscommunication, perhaps even saved by it. In the world of chemotherapy, it is the absurd that strikes the rule, not the logical. It is the clown that saves the party, not the cake. It is the ridiculous that sobers us, not the solemn.

During each of the many difficult times of Marthy's treatment, we were able to maintain our sense of humor and our equilibrium because we didn't allow the unexpected to knock us off our emotional feet. Visualizations can be most useful when trying to maintain balance and perspective. The two images I like and use most are what I call "becoming an umbrella" and "the rock on the beach."

In "becoming an umbrella," I visualize myself with an umbrella over my shoulder. Everything said or done to me that I don't like I allow to strike the umbrella and simply slide off. None of it sticks to me. None of it reaches me.

When I become "a rock on the beach," I see approaching challenges as waves advancing on my beach. I'm a rock on that beach and I've the choice to either breast the waves, attempt to bar their advance, or simply stand and let them slide by without affecting me.

Marthy likes to use either of two visualizations she calls "the pond" and "the beach." No matter how tumultuous the world may storm around her pond, she remains still and calm and without ripples. Or when she is feeling most disrupted emotionally, she can visualize herself lying on a sandy beach with warm little waves washing around her feet. I asked if she used either of them the night she awoke to find herself covered in blood.

"The pond, of course," she said. "I had one right in my lap."

You can create your own images, places, or analogies that work to help you remain in the eye of the hurricane while all around you is tossed and torn. Don't allow yourself to be caught in the fringes of the storms; remain in the center and you'll remain calm. From this position you can see clearly while others around you are blinded by the tempest. Above all, when life's challenges are most severe, remember to breathe. Look around yourself and you'll realize you are stable, steady on your feet and able to make calm decisions.

Marthy's color was red. What's your color?

EXERCISES FOR CHAPTER EIGHTEEN

Sit quietly in a busy location and feel the storm around you.

Take long breaths; feel your center.

Open your emotional umbrella.

Close your eyes and feel like a rock.

Carry a favorite stone in your pocket to remind you.

Never pick up anything bigger than a bowling ball without
expecting a hernia.

Chapter Nineteen
Blackberry Battles

I was living alone in Issaquah, Washington, when my sister began to lose her battle with lymphoma. I had purchased a large house on the side of Squak Mountain and was in the process of fixing the place up—a catharsis that I hoped would heal me of my grief over losing our brother Christopher. But I hadn't done my homework and the decision to choose Issaquah had been made out of pure nostalgia.

My father had loved Issaquah. When I was a child, we used to stop there on our way to anywhere east of the Cascades. But for all its mountainous beauty, Issaquah is not a location suitable for losing a case of melancholy. Seattle enjoys a lot of rain and even more gray days when it could have rained. Issaquah enjoys a full sixty percent more precipitation than Seattle. I should have known by the end of the first week when I realized I was one of only a handful who owned a convertible.

In preparation for the renovation of the house, I either gave away or sold much of my furniture and stashed the rest in a storage unit in West Seattle. I remember rattling around inside my new four-level home, driving to Portland every week to spend three or four days with my sister, and returning to pace among the echoes of my empty home alone in the rain.

I slept on the top floor overlooking a deeply wooded ravine—steep and green and wet. Here, in my grandmother's brass bed, my sister used to sleep when she came to visit. She claimed she got the best night's sleep there, high over my forested gorge in what she called "the tree-house room." In this room, I began to sleep late on the days I remained in Issaquah, rising only to eat or wander aimlessly about the empty house. All the floors were made of finely finished oak, smooth and cold, and I couldn't walk about them barefoot without my nose beginning to run. So I spent that winter alone: a sad, runny-nosed, barefoot man pacing about a large empty house.

In the spring, a pair of varied thrushes built their nest in the top of a cedar just beyond my window. I watched them build it, then sit upon it, then feed and raise a family in it. To this day, the sole note of a varied thrush brings upon a most singular melancholy, which harkens back to my days of despair on the side of Squak Mountain.

As my sister sank, I sank also. By August I was so low I could barely find my way to the bathroom. The days I spent at my sister's home in northwest Portland, I was jovial and supportive, reassuring her that her lymphoma was nothing like the one that had taken our little brother. She listened to me patiently, I realize now, understanding my need to deny her impending death.

I joked. I sang old family songs. I told her fibs about working on my house in Issaquah. Then, I would return to lie in my bed in the tree-house room and watch the varied thrushes. An odd anger began to well up within me. I wanted to strike back at a Universe that would make my sister suffer. The same Universe that had dismissed my brother, Christopher, so summarily was now taking her, too. Someone needed to be punished; that much was clear. I didn't realize it was myself I wanted to hurt.

I became so angry that if I could have gotten my hands around God's throat, I'd have ended it for all of us.

One morning, late with the gray high and light in the sky, I noticed from my tree-house window that a fringe of blackberries had crept up the ravine and into my front yard. I remembered that when I was a child, I would lie in my room above a chestnut tree and listen to my father pull Scotch broom from our fields until the small hours of the morning when I could no longer keep my eyes open. I had wondered then why he worked so hard in the fields so late into the night. I didn't understand his escape until much later, when my mother divorced him. I watched him shake his head in bewilderment and go out into the fields, calling the dogs, the flashlight on his head bobbing into a sea of Scotch broom. High in my bedroom in Issaquah, I finally understood that my father vented his frustrations on the hapless broom under the guise of clearing the fields. He'd cleared several acres by hand by the time they divorced.

I had no Scotch broom on my Squak Mountain acre above Issaquah, but there were those encroaching blackberries. I climbed out of bed and ran down two flights to the workroom to unbury my old machete.

I battled blackberries for four hours that day. Resting on the deck afterward, I realized I felt better than I had in months—strangely purged and oddly cleansed by the exercise. I was dirty and sore and scratched in several places. I felt an inexplicable satisfaction while examining the blood that had dried on my arms and legs. Now I understand that a large part of that peculiar satisfaction involved allowing the blackberries to punish me, but I would have denied it then. I believed I simply needed to play god and exercise control over something's life. If I couldn't control my sister's destiny, the blackberries' fate would have to do.

I know a woman who developed an enormous anger towards her cancer. She had trouble sleeping every night, which only exacerbated the side effects of the chemotherapy. On the advice of her therapist, she bought a large, heavy punching bag and hung it in the garage. On the nights when she couldn't sleep, her husband could hear her in the garage slugging it out with the Universe. Her exercise helped her maintain a positive attitude during her treatment and she also developed a mean left hook. You never know when either of those will come in handy.

We all need to express our frustrations at times. Venting spleen in a productive manner can only be healthy for us. My grandmother Reed used to quote an old adage: Hate is an acid that harms the vessel in which it's stored more than the person on whom it's poured. When you hate someone or something specifically, it's easy to pour your acid on them and be rid of it. When you hate what's happening to you, there's nothing to get your hands on, no one to scream at, and no one to blame but yourself.

Don't beat yourself up. Let the blackberries do it. Buy a machete and find a clump of berries. Or hang up a punching bag. Chop kindling. Beat a rug.

Whatever you find you can enjoy, use it to take a swing at the Universe. The Cosmos can take it. Universes don't hold grudges. They're much bigger than that.

Exercises for Chapter Nineteen

Find a clump of blackberry bushes to whack.

If you can't find any blackberries, weed your garden.

If you haven't got a garden, buy a punching bag.

If you haven't got a punching bag, take a swing at your pillow.

Chapter Twenty

Listen to Your Patient, Listen to Yourself

Sometimes in the heat of battle, we can become so caught up in our resistance that we forget to look around and check our position. Sometimes, when we act out of instinct instead of with thoughtful consideration, we find ourselves deep in enemy territory, accomplishing the opposite of what we intend.

An acquaintance of mine related a story about her husband learning to accept her cancer and chemotherapy. When she began to lose her hair during treatment, her husband admonished her to always wear a wig or a hat. She assumed he found her hair loss unattractive. She was hurt and recoiled from a confrontation with him, never asking why he insisted she cover her head. She wasn't comfortable wearing wigs but developed the habit of covering her scalp with a baseball cap, just to accommodate him. Her friends pitched in and soon she had a wide collection of caps from which to choose.

One night at a party with friends, she forgot to wear her cap to the dinner table.

"Go get your hat," her husband whispered.

"I can't just get up in the middle of the meal and come back with a hat on," she whispered back.

"If you don't, I'll go get it and bring it to you," he replied.

He so upset her that she burst into tears and left the table. A couple of her friends followed her to a family room away from the party. There they coaxed from her the cause of her tears. Together, they coated her head with water-soluble glue left over from a child's school-project. Then they trimmed the tail of the family poodle and thatched the top of her head with a ragged toupee of black fur. She returned to the dinner table and was greeted by an uproar of laughter, including her husband's.

This opened communication between them regarding why he was uncomfortable when she appeared uncovered. She discovered that it wasn't because he found her unattractive but because the loss of hair posed a constant reminder that his beloved was at risk. She realized then that he had not been reading the materials and books that she brought home from the clinic. Neither had he discussed her treatments with any of her doctors. Her primary caregiver, though far from finding her unattractive, had slipped into a denial of his loved one's condition out of self-preservation.

The problem is that denial doesn't preserve anyone. Instead it preserves fear. And fear is the killer, not cancer. Fear can kill a relationship just when that relationship may present the only quality of life left for a couple.

So what kills fear? Communication and humor kill fear.

Never be afraid to talk about your fears. Never think that you must protect a patient or a caregiver by not saying the things that keep you awake late at night. He or she probably needs to talk to you about the same things. And never, ever be afraid to laugh at your fears. Laughter dissolves fear like sunshine dispels darkness.

EXERCISES FOR CHAPTER TWENTY

Ask your patient a question a day.

Listen to the answer.

Remind your patient that bald is beautiful.

Be kind to poodles; you never know when you'll need one.

Chapter Twenty-one
Hurrying Off to Nowhere

I overslept today. When I woke I had barely enough time to dress, grab my briefcase, and beat my way to the dock in time to catch the 8:45 ferry. I didn't warm up my car enough; it ran crankily all morning.

I brushed a kiss by Marthy and flew out the door. A familiar anxiety blossomed in my chest. I tailgated an old pick-up truck that dawdled up the highway ahead of me as if I was going to be late to something very important, something that could not happen without me. Of course, the ferry would still have left had I not made the dock in time. I doubt the captain or first mate or even a single deck hand would have noticed my absence. And what would I have missed? Just a ferry. That's all. I would have had to wait fifty-five minutes for the 9:40 ferry.

But I made the 8:45 and sat and chatted with Lois Shigley on the passenger deck, drinking black coffee on an empty stomach, a sure way to relax that familiar anxiety-rush.

"Did you see that guy in the pick-up?" she asked me. "I thought we were never going to make this boat."

"I was right behind him," I said. "He was only doing thirty-five in the fifty zone. I'd have passed him but after we leave town, I think we're all in line for the ferry and I don't like to cut in front of people."

"I know what you mean," she said, "but he wasn't even going for the ferry. He pulled off half a mile up the hill. He must have known he was holding us up—he had a dozen cars lined up so close behind him that it looked like he had a magnet on his bumper."

When we reached Seattle, I called Marthy to brag about my achievement—making the ferry in twelve minutes flat. She told me the client I'd been hurrying to meet had called and asked that I call him before coming to his office. I called him. The materials he'd been preparing for me were not ready: could I come by just after lunch instead? He'd tried to reach me before I left to catch the ferry but had just missed me as I rushed out of the house. Now I was three hours early.

Marthy had finished eleven months of chemotherapy a week before. I had not felt rushed at any time during her treatment, not even when I was late for a ferry or for a doctor's appointment. While Marthy was in treatment, I'd felt a pace imposed upon me, a peaceful pace, one in keeping with whatever step the Universe demanded of us. Whatever it took, I was committed to Marthy's treatment and I knew the most wholesome and successful way to attack a cancer was to reduce the stress in one's life. No anxieties, no worries, no fears. Keep your goals in sight. Focus on the positive and remember to breathe.

Then the treatments were over and the real time began again. Real time with what seemed like real problems, like making a living and making time for work, each other, families, and friends. And making ferries. Suddenly the pace seemed to have accelerated for us. No more lazy mornings lying in each other's arms, sharing our dreams and watching the early birds at our feeders. Now each minute of the day had to be productive. Why the change?

There were no exams to see if Marthy had passed the test of chemotherapy. No x-rays, no blood counts, no true-false or multiple-choice quiz to prove she'd beaten her cancer. We couldn't open the door to see if the monster was gone; we simply had to sit and wait for his knock to know if he was still there. And not hearing a knock wasn't necessarily proof of anything except that he hadn't knocked yet. We were expected, without looking to see, to pick up our lives and get on with them as if there was no monster at the door. So we hurried to get things done before it knocked, just as if we were preparing for a visitor but weren't sure when, or even if, to expect it. Of course, we tried hard not to expect it but found ourselves listening over our shoulders every minute, waiting and wondering.

Suddenly I was in a hurry. A hurry to get on with it, make the decisions, make a living, make time for everyone (especially Marthy), make all this happen before the monster knocked on the door. Make those ferries. Or what? Or miss them. God help us if I missed a ferry. If I missed a ferry, I might miss a decision. Maybe the monster might knock.

The morning I made the 8:45 in twelve minutes flat, but unexpectedly found myself with three hours to spare, I sat in a café and ate a leisurely breakfast, ruminating in both definitions of the word. I remembered that while my little brother was considered to be in remission, he had adopted a poem by Robert Frost. It is titled "The Secret." It speaks of people metaphorically standing around a situation and supposing about it, while the Secret itself simply sits in the center and knows.

I also recalled an old Western song I had printed out for my brother during this period. I had sealed it in plastic and provided it with a hook for the showerhead so he could sing it each morning while bathing. He later reminded me that his uncorrected vision was 20/500 and that he rarely wore his glasses in the shower. The song spoke of loving like you've never been hurt and dancing like nobody is watching you, essentially, living life for the simple sake of living.

I don't guess that he had any country twang at heart because, to the best of my knowledge, he never sang a word of that song. But I was sure I knew what he had to do to beat his cancer and was in a hurry to give him the benefit of my knowledge. The more I pushed the song on him, the more he resisted it. I learned then that no one can tell anyone else how to do anything so personal as live. All we can do is remind ourselves not to be in a hurry to get nowhere.

Take a breath. Don't worry about singing or whether you do or don't need the money. Forget all the advice your loved ones give you. Don't hurry to make a ferry, and don't let anyone hurry you.

Above all, don't follow anyone else's example. Set one.

EXERCISES FOR CHAPTER TWENTY-ONE

If you find yourself hurried, stop and make yourself late.

Think of someplace you should go today and then sit in the sun instead.

Don't do any of the exercises in this book if you don't want to.

Chapter Twenty-two
No Justice, No Paybacks

I'm reminded of one of my earliest favorite poems. By that I mean that as I age, I find I have more and more favorite poems, very few of them written by myself, sadly. It became my favorite when I was a young college student taking too many poetry and literature classes. I was unaware then that I would not be able to escape the pathos that is the bitter-sweet of life. The poem was called "A Man Said to the Universe," and it was written by Stephen Crane. In it, Crane speaks of having the courage to confront the Universe, only to discover that the Universe doesn't particularly care about our courage.

Yes, we're here. We exist. But our existence is fragile indeed. Just as the Universe has no obligation to us, our obligation is not to the Universe but to ourselves, or perhaps to one another. Our commitment is to pursue a good and happy life. To fulfill that obligation, we have to be ready to seek out the humor in every situation, no matter how bleak, no matter how tragic. A tough assignment, one rife with bloodied noses, but no one ever promised you a nose garden.

Don't expect any justice from the natural world. Justice is a construct created by humanity for the sole purpose of controlling our masses. Ask a fawn how fair a shake it feels the Universe has given it when wolves pull it down before its first spring. Ask my brother's daughter, who never had a chance to know her father. Or ask Marthy, whose son, Chris, was killed by a drunk driver. No, don't look for justice in the natural world. If you want justice, read a romance novel or watch a made-for-television movie. Sometimes, you can find it in our courts, but not often even there.

Don't expect paybacks either. There is no balance sheet that will recompense you for all the good you do another. There are no rewards for being a caregiver—other than the rewards you give yourself.

We who are caregivers do so for one reason only. We need to contribute to the battle in some way. We hope to make a difference, perhaps provide the extra edge it will take to stem the tide. And sometimes we do. Sometimes all we hope for comes true. Sometimes it doesn't. But either way, we've done our best.

I know from experience that the worst thing one can feel, worse than even the most abject grief, is guilt. Guilt for not having done something, anything, to help that might have made the difference and saved the patient. If we don't try, we'll never know if we could have made the difference. In truth, the one we really save with our caregiving is ourself.

My sister, Karen, understood this more than anyone. She actively participated in the care of our brother as he fought his lymphoma. She held his head as he vomited, rubbed his feet when they ached, cooked and cleaned for him, and reassured him when he fought his fears. Four years after his death, she found a lump in her right breast.

"Not to worry," she said the day she drove to Seattle to tell me in person. "This is not a replay of Christopher's experience. This is breast cancer, something we can treat successfully."

She was wrong. The lump turned out to be metastasized lymphoma from her right armpit. The lymphoma was the same type that had taken Chris. A year later it took her also. Christopher had one benefit in his battle that she did not have. He had naiveté. He didn't know what to expect and so had less to fear. Karen knew too much.

She had fought so hard to save our brother that to find herself in the same fight again, this time for herself, hardly seemed fair. Everyone said so. Karen hated to hear it.

"Don't look for fair," she said. "Fair is where you go to ride Ferris wheels and eat cotton candy."

Don't let your patient ask, "Why me?" There is no answer to that question, at least not one we can discern in this lifetime. Ask only questions you can answer if you want to save your patient.

Marthy and I have a friend who called to say she'd just been diagnosed with breast cancer. Since she knew Marthy was battling something similar, she asked if we could come by to talk to her about what to expect.

We stopped by her house the next afternoon. Marthy was prepared to reassure the woman, advise her regarding what to look for in a physician, consider the options regarding lumpectomies versus partial versus radical mastectomies. She was not prepared for what awaited.

"Why me?" her friend lamented. "I'm young! I've got a husband and children. It's not fair!"

I still wonder at how self-absorbed a person must be to ask another with cancer to explain why he or she should have it and someone else should not. Marthy was offended. Our visit was brief. The friend didn't want answers to questions that might help her, only to feel sorry for herself. We could tell by the weary demeanor of her husband and children that she'd already worn out her only other witnesses. That's why she called Marthy.

As we left, Marthy turned to me with tears in her eyes.

"She's not going to make it," she said, "unless she loses that victim attitude."

Don't allow your patient to sink into the morass of self-pity. Don't let your patient ask, "Why me?" Help your patient realize the growth and strength and love and appreciation and all the rest of the great good that can come of meeting and surmounting a life-threatening challenge.

When I ask chemotherapy patients if they have one message they would pass on to any other person in the same straits, they all say the same thing, "Once you come through it, you'll never be the same again." And you'll never want to be like you were before the experience.

Focus your patient on what is to be gained, not what can be lost. Help him or her learn and grow from the experience. Embrace all that is good in it and discard the bad. Chemotherapy offers a chance not only to live, but to appreciate living in ways you could never have known before.

EXERCISES FOR CHAPTER TWENTY-TWO

Help your patient write, "Why not me?" a hundred times.

Write down all the reasons you feel privileged.

Exercise a privilege every day.

Practice clicking your heels.

Chapter Twenty-three

You Can't Dig Clams at High Tide

I grew up on an island. Inhabitants of islands are perhaps more sensitive to the cycles of nature than those who live in cities. I can't imagine anyone in the Bronx waking up in the morning and worrying that an unusually high tide had floated their boat and buoy away. Or someone in Duluth taking a day off just because the lowest tide of the year occurred in the middle of the workweek. Rural communities must be attuned to the weather and the seasons; they must live within the simple framework that nature provides.

When I was a child I learned three simple island rules. As I grew older, I discovered these rules applied to every endeavor I attempted. The rules are as follows:

1. You can't dig clams at high tide;
2. You can't drag the boat out at low tide; and
3. You can't bring back the ferry after you've missed it (although I did see one return to pick up the captain, who'd been left on the dock, but that's a totally different rule).

When my little brother was first diagnosed with his lymphoma, we made a pact to not leave any stone unturned in the pursuit of a successful treatment. As the years passed and treatment after treatment failed, we realized his was a losing battle. We did our best, but our best simply wasn't enough. When he was saying his final goodbyes, he mentioned he understood that some things just weren't meant to be. Months after his death, I realized we'd been violating all the rules of island life. We had tried to deny the tide of his destiny. Once his ferry had sailed, we tried to drag it back. He would have laughed at my interpretations, but he wouldn't have denied them.

Please don't misunderstand my story. I would never advocate that anyone should not try to his or her utmost to defeat a cancer. I'm only reminding you, as caregivers, that sometimes you can't win. This applies not only to your biggest battle, but to every day of chemotherapy as well.

You wouldn't drag a friend with the flu out to dinner. Don't force a patient to go out if he or she isn't feeling well. I once thought forcing my brother to go out with friends would lift his spirits. He gave in and went with me in spite of his disinclination. Several close friends met us at a nearby Thai restaurant, where we watched him throw up repeatedly into his plate. As his plate filled, I pleaded with the waitress to bring us a bowl. She responded by bringing a teacup. Each of us then provided our plates in turn until he had filled them all. Not so oddly, the dinner and the evening became abbreviated. No one had much of an appetite.

On a day when my stepfather, Ed, was at his lowest, both physically and emotionally, I thought I'd lift his spirits with some humor. I teased him about something inconsequential that I don't remember now, though I'll never forget his response. He shouted at me in anger. I explained I was only trying to cheer him up.

"I don't want to be cheered up," he said. "I'm not happy and I don't want to be happy! People don't always have to be happy!"

Don't try to force your patient to be cheerful. There are times when a patient needs to feel miserable because he or she indeed does feel miserable. You can offer an opportunity to look on the bright side—point out the first robin of spring or the first crocus—but don't insist that he or she appreciate it. Chemotherapy is not about you or wanting your patient to feel better. Chemotherapy is about feeling miserable and sometimes that's just what he or she has to do.

You shouldn't always listen to your patient, either. Pay attention to the signs of chemotherapy and look for the openings. Marthy and I tried to do something fun on the days we had to go to Seattle for her treatments. We'd take ourselves out to breakfast on the way to her appointments or to lunch after, and then a movie or just poking about antique shops or museums. As her treatments wore on and she wore out, she insisted we continue our "little get-aways," as she called them. But I could see the fatigue in her eyes, the emptiness that chemotherapy brings to a patient, and a total lack of reserves. I'd tell her I thought we'd better get back to the island.

"Let's just head for the ferry," I'd say. "If you feel well enough when we get there, we can poke about West Seattle or have lunch."

She'd agree and we'd start the drive back to Fauntleroy and the ferry dock. By the time we'd hit Spokane Street she'd be asleep in the front seat. She was constantly worrying that she'd become a burden to me and that her chemotherapy would inconvenience me. I just as constantly reassured her that there was nothing more I'd rather do than drive around with her sleeping alongside me.

Of course chemotherapy is an imposition. Cancer is the greatest imposition of all, and its treatment and cure cannot be of any less magnitude. Of course Marthy's chemotherapy inconvenienced me. I wanted to be inconvenienced if she was to be under treatment. I wanted to take care of her, to do whatever I could to help, and to continue to share our lives together. That's what a caregiver wants and that's what a caregiver does.

Pick your spots. Pay attention to the tides of chemotherapy. Don't try to drag the boat out at low tide; it will only become mired in the mud, and you're likely to wreck your back and your best sneakers too. And don't try to dig clams at high tide. In Puget Sound the tides vary as much as fifteen feet, and most of us cannot wield a shovel well while under water and holding our breath.

If the ferry has sailed, all you can do is sit on the dock and wave good-bye. Remember to breathe. Remember to focus on all you have accomplished and the importance of the treasures of your memories.

Never forget that every ending is a beginning. Your ferry will be coming along soon enough, too. Even if you have to spend a cold night in your car and wait until another morning. One ferry missed means another is met, and the far shore will always be waiting.

EXERCISES FOR CHAPTER TWENTY-THREE

Take your patient on a ferry ride.

Take your patient out for steamed clams (they come in a bucket).

Remind your patient that this will be a year to remember.

Chapter Twenty-four
Listening to the Music

Joseph Campbell once said he believed that the only real sin of living was that of inadvertence, of not paying attention to what's happening around you as you pass through. I interpret that as listening to the music.

A friend who needed a lumpectomy was referred to a highly respected female surgeon for the procedure. Nancy was frightened and in a hurry to respond to her diagnosis of cancer. She didn't feel she could afford the time it takes to seek a second opinion and was also reassured to have a woman doctor. She assumed a female surgeon would naturally be more sensitive to female issues such as breast cancer.

Nancy's husband had been a tremendous support and accompanied her to all her doctor appointments. When she first visited her surgeon's office, she went into the examination room alone, leaving her husband reading magazines in the waiting area.

Her female doctor entered and frowned.

"Let me guess," she said. "That would be your husband out in the waiting room."

"Why, yes, it is," Nancy answered, expecting a compliment for her husband to come next.

"I've got several like you who bring in their husbands," the surgeon rolled her eyes. "I don't know what it is with you women that you have to have so much help."

Nancy was stunned. She very nearly changed doctors right then, but was fearful of the delays. Her surgery was performed without complications but when she returned to have fluids drained from her surgical site, she again ran into the doctor's scowl.

When the physician brandished a syringe the size of the Chrysler Building, Nancy flinched. The doctor shook her head and plunged the syringe into Nancy's breast, much as though she was throwing darts.

Nancy gasped as the needle penetrated her.

The doctor hesitated.

"Are you all right?" she asked.

"I guess so," my friend replied timidly.

"Well, I'm only interested in you when you're *not* all right," the physician said and continued to withdraw the fluid.

I wonder if Nancy's surgeon ever read Joseph Campbell. As a caregiver, pay attention not only to your patient, but to those who provide treatment to your patient. Don't be afraid to speak up if anyone, even a doctor (especially if it's a doctor), appears insensitive to your patient.

My friend, Beth, was in the hospital for the last time. Her doctors had delivered their final diagnosis and left her to make her peace with her family and faith. On the second day, the child of a close friend came into the room carrying a present. When Beth opened the box, she laughed out loud.

"Tap shoes," she said. "I've been taking lessons for a year with borrowed shoes. Now I've got my own shoes at last!"

Over the protestations of her family, husband, and nurses, she put them on, got out of bed, and tapped her way out of the room and down the hall, past the nurse's station and several astonished hospital personnel.

When she finished, she was so fatigued she had to be helped back to her room.

"It was worth it," her husband, Chuck, remembers now. "I've never seen her so happy. We laughed and laughed."

We caregivers find ourselves in positions that are unique in many ways, some of them quite positive. We can learn from our patients, our experiences with them, facing their dilemmas, their fears, and their destinies. We can achieve a perspective more sharply attuned to what is most valuable in this lifetime, but we have to pay attention.

Never hide from what your patient is experiencing. Never run from the pain, whether it is your patient's or your own. Face the wind. Feel the cold as well as the warmth. Embrace the experience. The music of life plays all around us. Only those with deaf ears stumble on, oblivious to the melodies. Those who can hear can't help but dance.

Remember the dance? Don't wait for your own call before you listen. Turn your head now, cock an ear, and feel the rhythms. Take that first step. Put your right foot in, put your right foot out, put your right foot in and you shake it all about. Do the hokey-pokey and you turn yourself around. That's what it's all about.

EXERCISES FOR CHAPTER TWENTY-FOUR

Write down something you've always been afraid to try.

Put your right foot out.

Shake it all about.

Turn yourself around.

Do it.

Chapter Twenty-five
Time as an Ally

Time is your ally, not your enemy. Time is not short or long or filled or empty or even of the essence. You can be in time or on time or out of time. You can choose to waste time or make time or make use of your own time or take somebody else's time.

Time is what you make of it. You can choose to see time as short or long, just as you choose to consider that a night out with a friend was either a fine time or a bad time.

A redwood can expect to live hundreds of years (if redwoods have expectations). The average life expectancy of modern Homo sapiens is seventy-eight years for a female and seventy-three years for a male. Lengths of life vary from elephants to microorganisms. It is hardly profound to tell you time is relative. We've been hearing it all our lives.

Consider that mayflies live only eighteen hours. Within this three-quarters of one revolution of this planet, those creatures must be born, grow up, mature, meet, date, select a mate, lay their eggs, make their individual peace, and do their famous dance before they die. Since their dance begins at dusk, each mayfly may see one sunrise or one sunset or both, but never another midnight. No mayfly will ever know its own progeny, let alone its grandchildren. No mayfly will ever know what it means to contemplate its own existence. No mayfly will ever regret missing a moon fall, writing a novel, or never having streaked a campus.

A minute for a mayfly may be like a month for us, and a month to us may be like a few years to a redwood. What do you suppose a tree's lifetime is in comparison to a mountain's? A mountain's to a planet's? A planet's to a solar system's? A solar system's to a galaxy's? A galaxy's to that of the Universe?

The entirety of life on this planet exists as briefly as the illumination of a single flash bulb in the darkness of the whole Universe, yet each of us struggles just as mightily to see our next minute, our next morning, month, year, or millennium. Time may be relative, but tomorrow morning is just as important no matter who or what we are.

Some years ago I had occasion to work on a Dodge commercial with Professor Irwin Corey, a comedian who used to be a regular on the television show *Laugh In*. I was in my mid-thirties then, brash and full of myself, and a cigarette smoker. During one of the breaks in filming, Corey approached me and tapped the cigarette pack in my shirt pocket.

"How old are you," he asked, "about thirty-five?"

"Exactly," I said, impressed by his guess.

"I used to smoke," he nodded at me. "When I was thirty-five, I didn't care if I lived to be seventy-six."

He shook his finger and screwed up his face much like he used to on the television show.

"Now that I'm seventy-five," he said, "making seventy-six is a much bigger deal."

I remembered that conversation the first time I ever heard someone comment on my stepfather's age as he weakened from his cancers. The speaker was a hospice nurse and should have known better.

"You've got to keep in mind," the nurse told me, "that he's lived a good, long life."

Ed was seventy-seven but he didn't think he'd lived long enough. He wanted to be seventy-eight, and then seventy-nine, and to continue living as long as he could. He confided that he didn't sign into the hospice program because he believed he had less than six months to live, but because it afforded him greater Medicare benefits. He considered the decision to be economical, not practical.

The first time my brother, Chris, was told by his doctors that he had little time left, he said that if he had his life to live over again, he'd have spent less time doing his research and more time with his family and friends. Shortly thereafter, he entered an experimental chemotherapy program that succeeded in preparing him for a bone marrow transplant. The transplant resulted in an apparent remission.

When he got out of the hospital, he didn't resign his position at Dartmouth to spend more time with his family and friends, but embarked upon another summer of research at the University of Washington's Marine Biological Laboratories in Friday Harbor, Washington. When he relapsed a few months later, Chris again expressed regret for spending so much time on his work rather than with his loved ones.

What is it that demands we scurry around trying to make the most of our time while we think we have a lot of it, but slows us to less productivity and greater appreciation the less we have? As a writer, I like to think that if I were told I had only a few months to live, I'd produce a much greater amount of material than I do now. From my observations of loved ones as they failed, I think the truth would be that I'd produce much less. I would discover that my writing means much less than spending time with my loved ones.

Knowing someone is at risk of death has one advantage that the cataclysmic loss of a loved one cannot offer. You have the time to say your good-byes, to talk about anything and everything you otherwise might have regretted never having had the chance to say.

My father died the night after he began to tell me something he said was important but would keep until he saw me next. I will always wonder what he meant to say.

Chris told me in his final days that "he who lives the longest is not necessarily the winner." He also repeated many times that "the only treasures you can take with you are memories." So we spent his final days making memories. And every minute was a month for us; every month, a year.

Any day could be our last. We don't contemplate this fact as often as we might because it would drive us crazy. We can't live our lives as though today will be our last, but neither can we ignore the fact that it could be true. Somehow, we have to strike a delicate balance between believing we're about to die and feeling certain we'll live forever. It shouldn't be any different for a chemotherapy patient, but it is.

A chemotherapy patient is staring into the hood of the Grim Reaper. The rest of us wonder if we might die in an automobile accident or in our sleep or of old age (whatever that is). We have the luxury of contemplating just how we'd like to go. Chemotherapy patients don't have the luxury of wondering. The axe that will likely take them hangs suspended over their heads.

Your job is to help your patient appreciate each and every day you share. No matter how short or long our time will be, Marthy and I see any time together as a gift. Time is truly our ally because we choose to use it any way we like. Some days we work and some days we don't. Some days we sleep later and some days we rise early. The one thing we don't do is regret not having done something we wanted to do together.

When time becomes your enemy, when you never seem to have enough time, or when you're always running out of time, is when you need to re-prioritize. Look around.

It's high time you begin finding the time to live.

Exercises for Chapter Twenty-five

Try to see the world for the first time every time you wake.

Think of those you know and consider who will be alive in a hundred years.

Take your patient somewhere he or she has never been.

Don't wear your watch today.

Chapter Twenty-six

When to Hang On, When to Let Go

Growing up on Vashon Island, a small rural community in the middle of Puget Sound between Seattle and Tacoma, I had an older sister, two younger brothers, and children of all ages living in homes within a few miles of my own. Most parents worked off-island; today we would be considered latch-key kids. Back then, we just considered ourselves lucky. We all played together, creating every fantasy existence a child's mind could conceive. We built tree houses, fern camps, cave camps, beach camps, and even a tower camp with a tin roof at the top of our water tower in the round reservoir.

We occupied ourselves in as many ways as we could imagine. Tarzan was one of our heroes, so a favorite activity was swinging on a rope hung high in a tree. In the summers, we swung out over the Sound, yodeling like ape-men. Casting off from a tall clay cliff, the timing of our release over the water was not critical. We'd try to let go at the apex of the arc, of course, allowing us the longest drop into the deepest water, but if we timed our release badly, the worst that could happened was a shorter drop—a less than graceful fall, to the merriment of our friends.

Summers in the Pacific Northwest are short, and in cooler temperatures than August afforded, we played on a rope hung high in a huge madrone above a steep ravine. The rope crossed a gully filled with blackberries and all the other accouterments of terra firma, including rocks and roots and sharp branches, none as forgiving a landing pad as water. Here, the timing of our release took on added import, for if we didn't let go at the apex of the arc, we wouldn't land on the other side of the ravine, but rather in it. Here, the object of the swing was not to fall the longest distance, but the reverse—not to fall at all. The best of swings and timing would land us with one foot on a large root and one hand on a branch, safely up the far side of the ravine. Some of us appeared to be naturally adept at this practice, while others were not so adept.

I learned then that knowing when to hang on and when to let go was vital to survival, and that to freeze without decision could not only be dangerous but embarrassing as well. To find oneself dangling fearfully at the end of the rope, as its motion slowly stopped high above the blackberries, was potentially more damaging to the ego than to our bare arms and legs when we finally had to drop. So we all became adept at this game, which proved as daring as we might become before our teens. All but one of us.

One boy—we called him Fid—seemed to always be the one to fail no matter what game he attempted. If we played "dodge 'em," he was always the easiest to hit with the ball. If we competed to see who could ride the farthest down the beach trail without crashing on our bikes, he was the one who crashed first and worst. When it came to the rope swing, we should have known better than to let him jump off the cliff.

He swung out like the best of us but he never let go. We shouted at him, told him to let go. But he froze, clinging to the rope, not like Tarzan but like a frightened monkey. He swung back, but not far enough to reach the edge from which he'd leaped. On his second sweep, he inexplicably let go at the worst possible moment and fell upside down and backward into the ravine.

The rest of us howled uncontrollably until he didn't emerge from the thickets. We found him writhing on his back in silent pain, his elbows driven through his upper arms. A couple of operations and casts later, Fid was back to play with us but we never let him swing over land again.

In a functional sense, his playmates became his caregivers from that day forward. Each of us watched over him and no matter what game we played, he learned to trust us to tell him when to hang on and when to let go. After he broke both elbows, he never trusted himself to know when to let go, and he wouldn't go out on a swing unless we promised to tell him.

Chemotherapy patients need caregivers to tell them when to hang on and when to let go. Marthy vowed to defeat her cancer in every way possible. She tried to exercise regularly, but sometimes she simply didn't have the strength. Even when she was wobbling from weakness, she'd try to go walking no matter what the weather.

"You can take a day off," I'd tell her. "It's pouring out."

"I need to exercise regularly," she'd say.

"You also need to reserve the energy you have left. You can take this one day off," I'd convince her.

She tried to eat only healthy foods, but once in a while she'd crave some chocolate.

"Go ahead," I'd tell her.

"But it's not good for me," she'd worry.

"Maybe not for your body," I would agree, "but a little chocolate is food for your soul."

Choosing to battle a cancer with chemotherapy is a kind of hanging on. Hanging on to life. Hanging on to those you love.

In such a battle, loved ones tend to hang on to the patient, too. Sometimes this kind of hanging on is good and necessary. Sometimes it's not good and is not only unnecessary, but also needlessly painful.

As my stepfather's end came closer, he called his son, Greg, who lived a continent away in Virginia, to fly home to say goodbye. As I have mentioned earlier, he neglected, however, to tell Greg the purpose of the visit.

Greg is a firefighter and a trained emergency medical technician. He's seen his share of tragedies but had little time to prepare for his father's death: Ed fell into a coma just five days after his arrival. We brought a hospital bed into the family room and took turns sitting with him. When Ed stopped breathing, we were both present, with my last remaining brother, Craig, on hand as well.

I saw Ed had passed away. I took his hand in mine and stroked his forehead. Knowing his greatest concern was for my mother's care, I thought to reassure him. His time had come and I wanted him to be able to let go as easily as possible.

"It's all right," I said to him, unsure if he could still hear me. "Mom will be okay. We're here to take care of her for you."

My stepbrother screamed, "No!" and began to perform cardiopulmonary resuscitation on his father.

I let go of Ed and pulled Greg back. At first he resisted, but then he relaxed into my arms.

"He has to let go," I told him, "and you've got to let him."

Greg shook his head wearily.

"You're right," he said. "But with all my training, my instincts are not to let him die."

Those are the same instincts we all feel when we see a loved one slipping away. Most times, if a loved one is in danger of dying, resuscitation and emergency care are appropriate. But when a patient is lingering, dwindling slowly away, the caregiver has to allow his or her loved one to choose when to let go, even reassure him or her that it's all right to do so.

As a caregiver for a chemotherapy patient, most of the time you'll be encouraging your patient to hang on and to fight, even if just for another day or another hour. At the same time, be aware that no caregiver can tell a patient when it's time to let go. When that time comes, the patient knows. All you can do is tell your patient it's all right when he or she does go.

My sister was lying on her deathbed just hours before she slipped away. I asked her if she wanted to talk about death, about what lay ahead for her.

"Yes," she said. "No one else will let me; no one wants to hear it."

My brother faced the same dilemma. No one in our family would address the possibility he might not survive his lymphoma, though the doctors had already told him there was nothing more they could do.

People who are dying need to confront it, talk about it, get it out in the light, and examine it, so that they can escape their fear of it. If their caregivers and loved ones show fear of it, how can they face it fearlessly alone?

Don't be afraid to look at death. Remember to listen to your patient, no matter what he or she wants to say. Whatever it is, it must be the most important thing in his or her life. It may be the last.

EXERCISES FOR CHAPTER TWENTY-SIX

Find a swing to swing on.

Practice letting go at the top of the arc.

Practice walking with crutches.

Chapter Twenty-seven

Trusting the Absence of Stairs

Life is largely a matter of having the faith to step off into empty space. No one promised us security when we came tumbling out of our mothers' wombs. We didn't have any other choice but to emerge into a much colder and more frightening environment than the one in which we began.

As we grew and matured, we learned to rely on our memory and senses. Most of us learned early that mothers could be trusted, that if dogs growled at us a nip usually followed, and that loud noises rarely brought pleasant surprises.

If you have been a caregiver for a chemotherapy patient, this base of accumulated knowledge was your library of reference—the place you went to seek answers to any of the many challenges you faced. But if you are a first-time caregiver, you'll discover that many of the answers you seek are not to be found in your experiential library. As you continue, you'll discover that many of those answers are not to be found anywhere, least of all in books like this one.

Giving care to a loved one who is facing possible death is largely a matter of making up the answers as you go.

My little brother was a developmental biologist and as such believed in nothing he couldn't quantify in some way. If he couldn't weigh, measure, poke, prod, or otherwise test something, it simply didn't exist for him. Although he was primarily a microbiologist, he studied all kinds of life and was considered one of a few complete naturalists in the world. In all of his research, he found no evidence of life after death and so could not come to believe in the possibility of one. As he failed in his battle with his lymphoma, he prepared for his own death with the same predilection.

"Ashes to ashes," he said. "I've lived a life I can be proud of and I've no regrets other than I'll miss those I love so much."

He faced his death not with hope but with quiet resignation. To have believed in something he couldn't prove would have weakened him in his own eyes. It would have forced him to admit that he needed hope to face what every living thing ultimately must confront. He was a strong man, a man true to his convictions right to his end. I won't say he died happily, but he died without fear.

I don't know if he was right or if he was wrong. What I do know is that he was right for himself and that's what he needed to be. I knew others who believed they were passing into another, higher realm when they died. Perhaps they were. Perhaps we all do. Whether we do or don't isn't what is important in this life. What we need here is to be consistent with whatever it is that we truly believe.

What my brother believed shouldn't matter to you, no matter how extensive his education and experience. Just as it shouldn't matter to you what I believe, or what Marthy, your friends, doctor, minister, neighbor, grocer, or mechanic believes. In order to be truly certain, you can't simply go along with someone else's beliefs. You must decide for yourself. By yourself.

Your patient must decide for him or herself, too. His or her beliefs are not your decision. It's not your job, or even your right, to interfere or influence what he or she thinks awaits when the time to leave this world arrives. It doesn't matter if you agree or disagree with his or her beliefs; in fact, this non-interference rule applies especially if you disagree.

Your patient must have the faith to be able to step off into space without your arm to catch him. We are all born alone, and we all die alone. No matter how many people surround us throughout our lives, this rule holds constant. No one ever dies with another, even if they lie down together and cease breathing simultaneously.

No one ever battles cancer with another either. Every cancer patient makes his or her stand alone. A chemotherapy patient may have a caregiver like yourself, one who is a constant companion throughout all the appointments and treatments and sleepless nights. A chemotherapy patient may even have several caregivers, but there is still only one patient. And no matter how much you love your patient, no matter how much you try, you are still only the caregiver.

Your patient must have the faith to step off into space with no guarantees that the treatments will cure his or her cancer. Faith not in a god who will accept him or her into heaven, but in him or herself, here and now. Your patient must know without a doubt that he or she can accept whatever lies ahead.

Marthy feared many things during her treatment. She feared nausea, weakness, infections, hair loss, and, with the Taxol, neuropathy and anaphylactic shock. Perhaps most of all, she feared becoming a burden to her loved ones. After the end of the therapy, she felt a tremendous lift and release. But we weren't prepared for the new fear she discovered once she'd completed her therapy.

"Suddenly I miss the past year," she told me one evening.

"What could you miss about chemotherapy?" I asked in astonishment.

"I miss being in treatment," she said. "Now all I can do is wait. At least then, I was doing something to fight the cancer. Now I'm a sitting duck."

I could see it in her eyes. Now that we'd beaten the monster back from her door, all we could do was sit inside and wait to see if it knocked again.

"You don't have to just sit and wait," I said, though I had no idea what she might be able to do.

"You're right," she said with inspiration. "I can continue the fight. I can take the fight to the cancer instead of waiting for it to come back."

And that's just what she's done. She has sought the advice of naturopathic doctors, of nutritionists, and of psychologists. She subscribed to health periodicals and reads everything she can on the subject. She changed her diet and returned to exercising regularly. She is actively pursuing the cancer on her own terms. And most importantly, she no longer feels like a victim who's sitting around waiting to be picked off. She believes she can beat it and most importantly, she believes in herself. You can help your patient believe, too.

Ask about your patient's fears. Help him or her examine each one. Dismantle each fear by breaking it down into separate components. Show your patient that he or she has already handled a lot of fearful things and has come through with flying colors. Remind him or her that nothing in life that's worth having seems to come easily.

Help your patient look forward to events that will mark the end of things that he or she fears. Plan celebrations for the end of your patient's chemotherapy, for the beginning of a new life, a life free of cancer and fear. Focus on being free, not only of cancer, but of fear.

Remember that just as when we entered this world, we really haven't any other choice but to carry on as best we can. Will we tumble out of this womb into something colder and more frightening? Perhaps. But perhaps it is something more wonderful than anything anyone can imagine.

As my sister lay dying, I asked her if she was frightened.

"No," she said. "It occurs to me that dying can't be any more awful or wonderful than being born."

EXERCISES FOR CHAPTER TWENTY-SEVEN

Make a list of your patient's accomplishments.

Enlist your patient's aid in overcoming your own fears.

Take your patient to visit a maternity ward at a nearby hospital.

Hold a newborn infant.

Chapter Twenty-eight
Life Is a Butterfly

An analogy I like is that life is like a butterfly. If a butterfly chanced to alight on your finger, would you try to grab it and hold it? Of course not. You know a butterfly is fragile. To grab a butterfly would be to crush it, to knock the dust from its wings and kill it. Butterflies must be appreciated, not possessed. Likewise, we have to be willing to observe our lives unfolding like butterflies, to gratefully accept the beauty around us and live within it without trying to possess it.

I went out for coffee early one morning. I was disappointed to find that the coffee shop didn't open until nine on Saturdays. I was out of beans and couldn't make my own at home. I drove up town to Nasia's Islander Restaurant, thinking I might find my friend Mac Browne who breakfasts there nearly every morning. He wasn't there, but the smell of fresh coffee and flapjacks forced me into a booth by the front window. My old friend Liz, the little sister of an even older friend, greeted me and took my order.

Nasia's pancakes overflow a steak platter, and I was only able to consume a third of one. As I was finishing my second cup of coffee, a bicycle person—who I've seen riding around the island—walked his cycle by the window. This man must live on the street or in some falling garage, I thought, due to the condition of his clothes and his lack of a regular bathing habits. His teeth were bad, his beard was never quite long or short or well kept, and his thick glasses were never clean enough not to obscure his vision, which effected a permanent squint.

Yet he was always smiling and always engaged in conversation (with either himself or whomever he found within earshot). When I passed him on the road in my car, he never failed to wave and give me the thumbs-up sign. I didn't feel privileged by his attentions, as I'd see him offer the same gesture to every automobile that passed. Crazy Gary, another Island character, always saluted cars with a middle finger.

"Do you know the name of that bicycle guy?" I asked Liz as she refilled my cup.

She looked at me sideways.

"You know him," she said. "That's Richard. From grade school, remember?"

"Little Dickey?" I asked incredulously. I remembered him as a bright, hyperactive little boy who was friendly with everyone he knew. He still was, I realized, remembering his ubiquitous thumbs up.

"Yeah," Liz said, raising an eyebrow. "Scary, isn't it?"

She's right. It's very scary to see where another's path has taken him. Especially if that other path results in living on the street in some altered twilight of reality. There, indeed, might go any of us except for the grace of the Universe and perhaps missing a couple of potholes little Dickey had hit head on.

It's true for all of us. Every day of our lives, we're presented with opportunities to turn one way or another, morally as well as physically—in our walks, drives, and decisions regarding careers, loves, or even where we might dine on any given evening. One turn might lead us to fame, fortune, gratification, and happy endings; another, as simple as answering a phone call versus letting it ring, could lead us to desperation, despair, an empty life, or an unhappy demise. What makes the difference? How can we tell which path leads to rewards and which will result in disaster?

This book does not pretend to divine the secrets of destiny. But I can tell you this: regardless of the turn that led little Dickey to grow up and live on his bicycle, Richard is happy. His teeth may be bad, his eyes may squint through dirty lenses, and he may forever need a bath, but he's still giving the thumbs up to the world with every pump of his pedals. The secret, then, is not to try to control your destiny, but to learn to accept it, no matter what it might bring.

Controlling one's destiny is virtually impossible anyway. Even if we eat a healthy diet, exercise regularly, save all our money, go to the right schools, and generally pursue a good and wholesome life, we can still be struck down by what insurance companies call an Act of God. Though we cannot control what happens to us, we can control how we respond to it. Of course, we've all heard this a thousand times. We hear it over and over for one simple reason: it's true.

Whatever has happened to little Dickey, he has chosen his response. He has chosen to ride his bicycle rather than drive a station wagon, convertible, or take the bus. No matter that you or I might have chosen an entirely different response, little Dickey's response was his and his alone. And though I could never live in the manner he has chosen, I have to admire his attitude. Because, when you stop to think about it, when everything in our lives is reduced to the most common of denominators, all we really can choose is our attitude. And, when it comes to attitude, our choices become even more limited. Thumbs up or thumbs down.

I used to tell my kids that everyone lives in the same field. If you're city folk, you can consider it the same city block or suburban development. The point is, this field is filled with all that life has to offer; some of it is clover and some of it is cow pies. As we walk through this field, we certainly want to be aware of the cow pies in order to avoid stepping in them, but we must also be aware of the clover. Some people pass through seeing only cow pies. Oddly enough, these people seem to step in more than most. Some people see only clover. Not so oddly, these people step in a few cow pies they didn't see coming, but at least they don't seem to mind it as much.

The best navigators can see the cow pies but focus on the clover. They sometimes flop down in the clover to idle an afternoon away by looking for four-leafs. And sometimes the best time to do that is just after you've stepped in a cow pie. The pursuit of a happy life is all about the same things that walking through a field without getting too dirty is all about. It's about paying attention and staying in balance. And balance is all about attitude.

Trying too hard to control your destiny is a little like tilling a field but gripping your tractor's steering wheel too tightly. Every farmer knows that the only way to steer a straight furrow is not to hold the wheel too tightly. As the front tires hit clods and rocks, they bounce this way and that. The steering wheel swings wildly with them, sometimes with great force. If you try to control it too firmly, the wheel will bruise your hands, wear your arms out, and perhaps break a thumb. The trick to tilling a straight furrow is to grip the wheel lightly, to gently guide the tractor in the desired direction while allowing the tires to jump and bump a little each way.

Life tosses us similarly back and forth, sometimes with thumb-breaking ferocity and most times beyond our control. As if in a plane on autopilot, we try to keep a general heading, but the wind and weather buffet us constantly—events swing us wildly off course for long moments at a time and maybe even spill our coffees in our laps. But then we correct and swerve back to our course, or often past it in over—correction. Cow pies or clover, farmers on tractors, pilots in airplanes, butterflies chancing to alight on your finger—you can think of many more analogies more appropriate for yourself. We, all of us, are simply trying to find our way through the labyrinths of our lives. But to what? What awaits us all at the end? We're all going to die. Is dying the point then? I don't think so.

I think the labyrinth is the point. Living to the best of our abilities. Regardless of your religion or lack of any, how you live must be more important than how long you live. Quality of life is the answer to any question, no matter who's asking it. That's why you're a caregiver. That's also why you're reading this book.

Take a breath. Feel good. Help your patient feel good. Find a way to laugh at any circumstance. Learn to dance when you hear the music. When you can't hear a tune, whistle one. This experience, the experiment of carbon-based existence on the third planet from the sun in but one solar system among so many scattered throughout the ever-expanding Universe, is singular indeed. It is singular to you. It's singular to your patient. It's singular to your family, your friends, neighbors, strangers, mice, birds, snakes, insects, trees, flowers, rocks, grains of sand, molecules of the air we breathe, sub-atomic particles accelerating right through us. The same rule applies to each and every one, whether we are rock, person, or tree.

Be here. Be present. Be happy.

Thumbs up.

EXERCISE FOR CHAPTER TWENTY-EIGHT

Give a thumbs-up to a stranger.

Postscript

Marthy completed eleven months of chemotherapy, and now this book seems oddly superfluous. When we think back on her year of chemotherapy, it appears to have happened quite a long time ago to another couple in another place. Reality, we've discovered, has much to do with the here and now, not the past.

A month after Marthy completed her chemotherapy, she went back to work. In the next few weeks she came down with a head cold, chest cold, stomach flu, and a bladder infection. I suggested that perhaps she had returned to work too soon, but she only laughed.

"You've no idea how good it feels to feel bad for normal reasons," she said.

One day on the ferry, I bumped into a friend who had recently completed chemotherapy also. She too was suffering from a severe cold. Her eyes were red and tearing, and her nose was red and running. She looked and sounded miserable.

I exhibited my usual tact.

"You look miserable," I said.

"I am," she said. "Isn't it wonderful? I've never felt so good with a lousy cold in my life."

She went on to say the same things Marthy has said regarding the end of her chemotherapy.

"I wouldn't have thought I'd ever say this," my friend confided. "But I miss being in chemotherapy."

Marthy tells me she found being in treatment easier and less stressful than getting on with her life afterward.

"It was easier to have faith in a doctor I trusted than in myself,"

Marthy said one evening. "When I was in chemotherapy, all I had to do was follow orders. Now I have to give the orders to myself. And I don't have as much confidence in my new boss."

Sporting a thick head of new hair, my friend on the ferry missed being as visible as only a bald woman can be.

"When I was bald, everyone knew what I was going through," she said. "The support was fantastic. Everywhere I went people encouraged me. Cancer survivors would come up and tell me wonderful success stories. It wasn't really sympathy, I think, but support. Definitely much more support than I get now. Now I'm expected to just get on with it. You know, be normal."

The problem is that cancer survivors will never be normal again. Their perspectives on everything are forever altered by the chemotherapy experience. Once their battle becomes less visible, we forget about them and go on about our own personal daily grinds. But their duel with cancer remains just as fresh as the day they were slapped in the face with the mailed glove of diagnosis.

"Now," Marthy tells me, "I have to take the fight to the cancer, wherever it is. I've got to come up with ways to be healthier all by myself."

Every little ache and pain she might have dismissed without a thought prior to her diagnosis is now suspect.

"I find myself wondering if it's coming back," she says.

An odd exhaustion settled on her several weeks after most of the chemicals should have cleared from her system. She had no stamina and no reserves once she became fatigued. She worried that her tiredness could be an early warning of relapse, that the cancer had silently metastasized to some other location within her.

I tried to reassure her. I told her that I thought it only logical that she would have little strength after nearly a year of chemotherapy.

"I need to know what it is," she insisted.

"If you have to have a label," I said, "then call it 'a non-specific malaise resulting from eleven months of immune system depression.'"

She laughed.

"Nice try," she said and looked up chemotherapy in our medical encyclopedia.

"What a relief," she said. "There's actually something called 'Post-chemotherapy Fatigue.' That's what's happening to me. It's nothing to worry about. It's normal."

When you are actively involved in a treatment protocol, you have a doctor and a clinical team to reassure you that certain symptoms are normal, or at least to be expected. When you are on your own, you must find your own labels and your own reassurance that all is unfolding as it should.

Remember: once a cancer patient, always a cancer patient. And, by the same token: once a caregiver, always a caregiver. The hardest part of treatment is always the wait, whether it's in the office before the diagnosis, before the injection, or before the radiation. And, especially, the wait after the active treatment ends.

The unknown is the common element and enemy. The unknown is always the worst fear. The monster is still outside your door, but you can't peek to see if it's there. All you can do is wait to see if it knocks again.

Don't let your patient cower inside. Go out and chase the monsters away. Help your patient take an active approach to remaining in remission. Waiting for things to happen to us is how we become victims. Don't wait. Make things happen and they'll turn out to be the right things.

You are, after all, the caregiver.

About the Author

Steve Reed is a professional writer and long-time caregiver. His caregiving experiences began when assumed responsibility for the care of his siblings, Chris and Karen, both of whom fell to lymphoma within one year of each other. After Karen died in 1994, Reed made plans to move back to his hometown of Vashon Island, Washington, to live on the family property where both of his siblings' ashes are scattered. While preparing the property, he re-met Marthy, who had been among his first friends when he arrived on the island at the age of seven. They had lost touch after high school, until they were reunited by what Terry Tempest Williams calls "the shared landscape of grief." While she was going through chemotherapy to treat breast cancer, Marthy asked Steve to write what has become *Pebbling the Walk*. Marthy and Steve now live together in a small cottage with a river stone fireplace in the woods on Vashon Island.

Steve Reed is a technical courseware designer for IBID Publishing, a columnist for *Northwest Prime Time News*, a contributor for *Beachcomber* and *The Ticket* (both weekly newspapers), and has written features for *Pacific Maritime Magazine*. This is his first published book of nonfiction.